MY CHILD
IS NOT
A
NUT ALLERGY

MY CHILD
IS NOT
A
NUT ALLERGY

A Practical Guide & Healing Journey from
Anaphylaxis to Wellness

BY

NATALIA ELDER

Published by Elderrat Publishers 2015
ABN 19789677583

A catalogue record for this book is available from the National Library of Australia.

Author Photo owned by author.
Book Cover Design and Original Graphics by Mitch Mottley
Formatting by Tim Edler
N.B. Some names have been changed to protect the innocent.
First Edition 2015

Publisher's Address:
Elderrat Publishers
P.O. Box 3385
Loganholme Queensland 4129
AUSTRALIA

Author Contacts:
Email: nataliaelder@outlook.com
Facebook Page: Facebook.com/my child is not a nut allergy
Website: www.nataliaelder.com

ISBN: (pbk) 978 – 0 – 9925554 – 0 - 5
(ebk) 978 – 0 – 9925554 – 1 - 2

DEDICATION

To my dearest mother, Edith who taught me patience, resilience and to use my intuition.

To my husband, Adam who always challenges me to be all that I am.

To my sons, Freddie and Victor who are my greatest teachers of unconditional love, compassion and wisdom.

To my brother, Luke Valais who has always believed in my talent as a writer and is my voluntary Script Editor. Hopefully, one year he'll be paid all the back pay he rightly deserves!

To my family and friends who always give me support, kindness and share their wisdom. You know who you are!

Thank you; Thank you; Thank you.

You can never have enough knowledge.

LONE WOLF

DISCLAIMER

All medical, homeopathic and naturopathic information is accurate at time of publication. The journey, advice and comments by the author belong to the author. Acting on the advice of the author is the reader's own choice. Due to the nature of the advice, it is subjective to the author's journey and may or may not be relevant or appropriate for the reader or person living with a nut allergy. Any advice followed is entered at own risk of the reader and/ or person experiencing anaphylactic reactions to nuts or any other type of life-threatening allergy. However, this book is written and shared with the utmost intention of support, compassion and wisdom for the good of all.

Go well. Stay healthy. Be happy.

Natalia Elder

CONTENTS

ACKNOWLEDGEMENTS

The prevalence of anaphylactic allergic reactions is now commonplace in the world. It seems everyone to whom I speak knows someone who has an anaphylactic allergy to a natural or synthetic substance.

All have been desperate for assistance in coping with living day-to-day with this affliction in the body, mind and spirit. Finding solutions to being part of the community and moving forward without fear is also a common issue. Ultimately, these parents want their children to grow up and lead happy, successful lives. They also want their families to be healed and maintain wellness.

When I let them know of our family's journey and that my son, Victor has healed himself from this life-threatening condition, they have urged me to put the information out there. Hence, "My Child Is Not A Nut Allergy" came into reality in the form of this book.

I'd like to acknowledge Endocrinologist and Author Deepak Chopra M.D. for his immense body of work in understanding the relationship of mind, body and spirit.

I'd also like to acknowledge Authors Louise L. Hay and Annette Noontil for their correlation between thoughts and illnesses that manifest in our bodies.

Thank you to Robyn Ehmen (nee Miller) for her generous assistance with healing Victor from anaphylactic reactions and getting the book published to help others with their healing process. I thank her for keeping me well, focused and fed whilst working on the book. I appreciate her validation in writing the book's Forward.

N.B. * * REMEMBER IT IS IMPERATIVE TO BE UNDER THE CARE OF HEALTH PROFESSIONALS AT ALL TIMES FOR SAFETY AND PEACE OF MIND DURING THE HEALING JOURNEY.

The Medical Profession and the Natural Therapies' Professions can and do work in harmony with each other when treating a person holistically.

Thank you to Robyn Ehmen and my brother, Luke for their generosity, wisdom and expertise when editing the book.
Thank you to my husband, Adam and my sons, Freddie and Victor for their support, patience and understanding - especially when I've needed help with household duties.

Natalia Elder

FORWARD

This is an amazing story of a journey of healing and self-discovery for a 15 year old boy called Victor. Victor's healing journey started with a severe anaphylactic, allergic reaction to nuts aged 7. Eight years later, he is free from all allergy signs and symptoms. Victor can eat all nuts and is a confident, well-adjusted and self-assured teenager.

Contact with nuts would cause Victor's face and air passages to swell up. He would stop breathing. This is called having an anaphylactic reaction. Medical first-aid involves the immediate use of the Epi-Pen Junior/ Epi-Pen (Australia) or Ana-Pen Junior/ Ana-Pen (New Zealand). Victor had to take his Epi-Pen to school and on all outings into the community. The Epi-Pen is an auto injector of Epinephrine (Adrenaline).

Victor's mother, Natalia showed great courage and determination to do everything she could to find a reason for her son's extreme allergy, as well as a solution, on the physical, emotional, mental and spiritual levels.

Natalia used everything that was available to help her son. Everyone was important in helping Victor: the local Doctor for first-aid intervention; the Allergy Specialist Doctor for finding out what exactly caused the anaphylactic reaction and providing an action plan for anaphylaxis (ascia); the Homeopath and the Naturopath for desensitising the nut allergy and giving advice on food selection; and the Chiropractor for keeping his skeleton in alignment whilst growing and developing.

This practical, self-help book guides you through the maze of caring for someone with a nut allergy. It's about managing the full constellation of family dynamics and integrating a child into school and community with confidence.

Natural Medicine offers gentle solutions to heal anaphylaxis and bring the whole child into balance. The Medical Profession saved Victor's life and gave him ways to prevent reoccurrence, but at this stage, they had no methods to heal his condition.

In Natural Medicine, the most important remedy for swelling of any kind, especially allergic swelling of the air passages, is Apis Mel. This is homeopathic bee venom. Bee venom causes tissue to swell. Therefore, homeopathic bee venom causes the swelling to go down. It works a treat! The other remedy for getting over the bad effects of certain foods is Nux Vom. These remedies can be obtained in low potency from the Health Food Store or higher potencies from a Homeopath/ Naturopath.

When consulting a Naturopathic Practitioner, allergies can be reduced by healing the gut which aids proper digestion of food. Food particles can leak through a damaged gut wall and cause an allergic response in the blood stream. After completing a gut repair, the remaining allergies can be desensitised. This involves the tiniest amounts of the offending foods taken under the tongue in droplet form. The dosage is gradually increased so that the immune system becomes balanced and a tolerance is achieved.

Sometimes, the immune and nervous systems can become set with responding abnormally to allergens. In this case, stimulation to acupressure points can bring about complete healing of the body. This technique was used on Victor and cleared all signs and symptoms of his nut and environmental allergies.

When Victor hit puberty, teenage moodiness and low self-esteem issues surfaced. Australian Bush Flower Essences proved effective to support his growth and development to maturity. Great results were obtained with the combination remedies called Abund and Confid. These can be purchased from a Health Food Store.

If allergies have impacted your life, you will find this a compelling read. The story is strategic and informative on all levels.

Robyn Ehmen R.N., N.D., Dip. Herbal Medicine, Dip. Counselling, Dip. Bowen Therapy
For all Natural Medicine Consultant and Treatment
In Australia, phone: 0411 055 687
Overseas, phone: +61 411 055 687
Email: proactive natural health@gmail.com

INTRODUCTION

'Childhood is meant to be a time of discovery and
freedom from responsibility.'

PIER 13

Remember when jumping off the pier was fun? There was no thought of
sharks or stingers in the water. No thought of breaking a bone or drowning.
No danger. Just pure unadulterated fun.

It was adults who first told us of the fears and dangers of
experiencing something new like jumping off a pier or climbing a tree.

As an adult, we know that there is a possibility of things going awry.
We want to protect our children from being hurt or dying because we love
them dearly.

When an anaphylactic reaction to nuts occurs out of the blue for no
apparent reason, one loses all understanding of the familiarity of learned
knowledge.

On June 15, 2005, my second-born son, Victor had a sudden, severe
reaction to eating Brazil nut chocolate. I remember feeling deeply in shock
and an overwhelming sense of foreboding and helplessness.

Luckily, my First Aid training had kicked in automatically. His face
half-swollen, his breathing wheezy and a red circle appearing on his throat
meant that his Epiglottis (a valve at back of the throat that allows food to
pass into the food pipe or air to pass into the wind pipe) was swollen.
Something dire was happening in his body. I had never seen an allergic
reaction before but I knew where the Epiglottis was and that if it swelled
enough, it would cut off his windpipe from the breath of life.

Being a practical person, I sat Victor down, calmed him and placed
an ice pack on his throat. I then rang the doctor's surgery for advice. The
receptionist told me to bring him there straight away.

Victor was seven years old. His nine and half year old brother,
Freddie was playing electronic games and his father, Adam was at work.

I packed up a stack of Freddie's favourite magazines and as calmly
as I could, bundled them into the car. It was a seven minute drive to the
doctor's surgery without traffic. School was out so it took longer. Forever. I
could see in the rear vision mirror that Victor was losing consciousness in
the back seat but I pressed on. Later, Freddie said that I drove like a racing
car driver. That one lesson I'd had in a race car over ten years ago at Surfer's
Paradise Raceway with my husband, Adam had paid off.

After I'd parked the car, I realised that I was another couple of minutes away from the doctor's surgery. Victor collapsed in the car park. I scooped him up and re-secured the ice pack on his throat.

I ran as fast as I could and asked Freddie to keep up. I remember dashing across the pedestrian crossing and passing a lady I knew from the football club. We said hellos and how are you, as you do, and replied with the usual fine pleasantries. How bizarre? I was running. Victor's life was in the balance. What if I'd said my son is dying? Would it have made any difference? Would she have heard me?

Frantic, I burst into the doctor's surgery and called out to the receptionist that my son couldn't breathe. A nurse appeared and immediately said, 'Follow me.'

Carried along by adrenaline alone, I walked briskly down the long corridor and followed the nurse without question. Glancing over my shoulder, I asked Freddie to sit outside and read his magazines, as I swung into the surgery and placed Victor on the bed. Barely conscious, the nurse stripped off his clothes and covered him with a white cotton blanket. With his white hair, I had a sudden déjà vu feeling of how he looked at birth.

Within moments, a doctor arrived. She immediately diagnosed that he'd had an anaphylactic reaction and gave him a shot of adrenaline, before slipping an oxygen mask over his nose and mouth. She said that we'd have to wait twenty minutes to see if he would return to normal. The doctor returned to her patients and the nurse remained with us. Adrenaline continued to pump through my body. I had no choice but to fight my worst fears and be there for my son.

His life hanging in the balance, I stayed with Victor hugging and stroking him, whispering words of love into his ear to keep him calm. The nurse said that he'd have a quicker reaction next time and to ring the paramedics, as there was less chance of survival.

I felt like my heart was in my throat, but I somehow detached myself from an adverse outcome. I stayed in the moment and went with the flow, as I had learnt through many years of spiritual growth, yoga and meditation.

After twenty minutes, the doctor returned and checked Victor's vital signs. Not happy, she gave him another adrenaline shot and continued with the oxygen therapy.

After another twenty minutes, Victor sat up. He was glowing in pure white light, like he was angelic or had had some sort of a rebirth (second chance at life). He pulled the mask off and smiled at me.
The doctor checked him over and said that he was fine to go. She said to take him home, feed him and return tomorrow for a check-up.

Relieved, I had managed to get Victor help in time to save his life. However, knowing that he was minutes away from death rocked me to the depth of my soul.

The well-meaning nurse, who gave me the candid statement of the hard truth that next time he may or may not survive, was a hefty dose of the reality and seriousness of his condition. I am forever grateful to the expertise of the doctor and nurse that saved his life.

Victor looked perfectly normal. He glowed with health and vitality after all that adrenaline and pure oxygen had been pumped into his cellular system. I knew though, inside his young body, that was not the case. Antibodies lay in wait to shut down his life force if it perceived an enemy attack by the next nut protein that neared or entered his body.

I felt we'd jumped off a pier into treacherous waters and we both didn't know how to swim. We were both sick to the stomach with fear, as the reality of the trauma set it.

Though Freddie knew what happened to Victor, he was unaware of the perils his brother was about to face and how it would impact on our family life.

Wrapping Victor in the blanket, I carried him back to the car on jelly-like legs. Somehow, I drove the car home.

Little did I know that there was worse to come? When my husband, Adam arrived home, he didn't believe me that Victor had a life-threatening condition. Victor looked well, more than well, he brimmed with vitality.

There wasn't time to ring Adam during the crisis and by the time I'd arrived home, I was exhausted and sick with shock and worry. How was I to proceed to take care of my family henceforth? There was no way of convincing Adam. A pragmatic person, he hadn't seen it with his own eyes. I realised then and there that I needed an immediate action plan.

IMMEDIATE ACTION PLAN

'Adversity is not a bad thing. It can make you aware of more important things that need attention in your life.'

THE 24 STEPS

1. FIRST AID

'Knowing the principles of First Aid gives one the tools for helping another human being before getting to professional health care for healing and survival.'

Immediately, I arranged for a doctor's appointment after first aid treatment to obtain 2 Epi-Pens (Self-administering syringe containing adrenaline). One was for home/ outing use and one was to be kept at kindergarten/ school.

The doctor also gave me a referral to an Allergy Specialist. She warned me that it could take three months or more to obtain an appointment, as there were very few practicing. 'As soon as you can,' she said, 'ring for an appointment.'

The next trip was to the Pharmacy. I asked the Pharmacist for the Epi-Pen Juniors/ Epi-Pens to have a year expiry date on them. N.B. ** Epi-Pens are expensive, (even though the government does offer some subsidiary). It saves money not having to return at shorter intervals for the First Aid item.

Just before the expiry date, I made a doctor's appointment to obtain new ones.

I handed in expired Epi-Pens to the Pharmacist for safe disposal, after using them to practice on oranges.

It was important that my child, my family and I knew how to use them.

N.B. ** CPR doesn't work on anaphylaxis. Locating the Epi-Pen Junior/ Epi-Pen, administering it and calling the paramedics are the only First Aid treatments. It may or may not work, but it's the best chance they have of staying alive, until they can get to hospital.

I asked the Pharmacist to show me how to use the Epi-Pen Junior. (Sometimes, they have a practice one under the counter.) These Epi-Pens came without adrenaline and needle, but they gave me a good feel of how they worked. I had read stories of how the adrenaline failed to be administered properly through inexperience or panic.

At home, I kept the Epi-Pen Junior/ Epi-Pen in the same place for quick and easy access along with his Personal Action Plan for Anaphylaxis. I kept mine in the linen cupboard centrally placed in the house. It was on a shelf so all the family could reach it, but it's not a place that's used very often and is out of sight. I didn't want my children to see it as a toy or curio object.

2. EDUCATION

'Knowledge provides an awareness and confidence to maintain health and live life well.'

Searching the internet for information on Nut Allergies was the next logical step. Most sites explained how the reaction occurred and gave valuable knowledge and advice.

To my surprise, I found that the nut protein was also in sesame seeds, E322, Hydrolysed Vegetable Protein, Soy Lecithin, blended oils and make-up.

There was also supporting evidence that by reintroducing the allergen in small amounts over a period of time, it may lessen and ultimately heal the nut allergy.

There was a website where you could purchase bracelets and pendants engraved with information that the wearer had a nut allergy. I decided against it. I feared that my child may be targeted and bullied at school because he was different. If another child didn't like him, they could easily give him some nuts/ nut product and unwittingly/ wittingly be rid of him for good!

I printed out all the information for reference and for the family to read. I then called a family conference to discuss the impact on the home and family. There were lots of questions and concerns.

I also printed out a copy for his school teachers, the office staff who usually deliver the First Aid and give out medication, and the Principal.

My child's Principal was unaware that the Epi-Pen Junior/ Epi-Pen was the only First Aid. They thought it was the paramedic's job to administer the Epi-Pen Junior/ Epi-Pen. They didn't realise that my child would be dead before paramedics arrived without the adrenaline shot.

That was seven years ago. Due to the increase in childhood anaphylactic reactions to allergens, teachers now have access to information from the government and are now trained in the usage of the Epi-Pen Junior/ Epi-Pen. It is also a part of all First Aid Courses.
Relief/ Supply Teachers also need to be informed of the child's nut allergy and First Aid treatment.

If possible, choose your child's teachers in Primary School. I found one teacher was a trained nurse and my child stayed in her multi-age class for three years. She had most of the children with allergies in her class and the whole class was taught about the signs and symptoms of an anaphylactic reaction. They were able to alert the teacher quickly if they noticed anyone having a reaction. All classroom colleagues were caring and supportive of my child. This allayed my fears somewhat and gave me a real sense that my child would be safe at school.

For special occasions, I gave the teacher a small stash of treats my child could eat. That way when other children brought in a cake, chocolates or lollies/ candy for their birthday, my child could celebrate too.

Some suggestions for treats are: Time Out Bars, Plain Chocolate, Kit-Kats, Freddos, Natural Lollies, Chips or Twisties.

Knowledge is a powerful thing, but it can also create more terror. Knowledge can prevent an anaphylactic reaction too and can help your child live a normal, healthy and happy life. I preferred to take on board the latter.

3. SPREAD THE WORD

'Keep your message simple and the whole world will understand it.'

The importance of alerting all people who came in immediate contact with my child was paramount.

I took time to speak with my extended family, friends, parents of your child's friends, teachers, children in their classroom, sporting & activity coaches, creative expression teachers (dance, instrument, art, and acting), school chaplain, nurse, P & C president, canteen convenor and religious leader. It was well worth the time. I considered it a necessity for the survival and welfare of my child, but it was also a great support to me and my family. To know that I wasn't alone in caring for my son 24/7 was tremendously therapeutic.

I explained to them all the ways of prevention; first aid treatment; and the absolute need to call the paramedics to transport Victor to hospital which would increase his chances of survival. Many people, to whom I spoke, knew someone with a nut allergy or other food allergy. (Be open to their suggestions and advice. Thank them kindly. Most people are caring and empathetic.) It was up to me, whether I took on board some, or all of their advice, but I always appreciated their consideration.

As a parent, I had taken on being my child's main carer. Having had other people willing to help and give me much needed breaks, was essential to my own health.

If people were willing to take Victor out, have them at their home for a few hours play with their child, or ultimately, have them for a sleep-over, it made it infinitely easier for my child to live a normal life in society.

By wrapping Victor in cotton wool, I realised wasn't doing him any favours. It would only make it harder later for him to socialise normally and to live an independent life in the real world.

I always expressed my gratitude to these wonderful, courageous and compassionate people who supported me unconditionally.

It was important to let them know that if an anaphylactic reaction occurred, I trusted them to perform First Aid and call the paramedics. That was the best thing they could do to help him. If it didn't work and Victor died, then I would have appreciated that they did everything in their power to save him.

After all, Victor could die if I was the First Aid Person.

4. FOOD LABELS

'Knowledge is power and calms the mind.'

Right from the get-go, I began to read labels of processed foods already in my pantry, fridge and freezer. I found it was essential to reduce the chances of accidental ingestion of nuts and nut traces.

I made a list of all the foods my child could or couldn't eat. N.B. *** I kept all the foods I already had. I had paid good money for them. The rest of my family still wanted to eat the foods that contain nuts or traces of nuts or foods processed on factory equipment.

It was imperative that my child could distinguish between foods he could or couldn't eat. Victor needed to know what their packaging looked like inside and outside of our home.

I taught Victor to read food labels. My child could read somewhat at seven. If he was younger, I would still have showed him them often, so that he could begin to recognise them by sight.

Most ingredients were obvious, if they were from nut origin. They would often be put in **bold letters** that the product may contain traces of nuts and/ or has been processed on factory equipment.

Some ingredients are not so obvious. For example:

- Amaretto - Almond Essence/ Liqueur
- Palm oil
- Blended oil - may contain oil from nuts
- Coconut - because it contains the word nut, it can be confusing to the child, so include it. Coconut is a drupe and not a true tree nut. It is also a fruit.
- Nutmeg - is a spice from the seed of a tropical tree. It also contains the word nut.
- Almond - is not a true nut. It is a drupe like the coconut. It is often in mixed nut products and people can become allergic to them.
- Soy Lecithin
- Hydrolysed Vegetable Protein
- E322 – Additive

5. A BALANCED DIET

'Since the dawn of time, Mother Nature has nurtured every living thing to thrive and survive.'

With considerable thought, I worked out a simple 'Daily Menu' for Victor. It included snacks of foods he liked to eat. He preferred to graze when hungry, than eat three set meals a day. I felt it was important to keep him happy and healthy. As he was still growing, he needed all the essential foods from the Five Food Groups.

Victor was a fussy eater. Sticking with mainly whole foods was the answer for him. During the week, I also worked outside the home, so including some processed foods was a necessity, especially for the school lunch box.

Initially, the canteen convenor said that my child wasn't allowed to eat at the canteen at all! I decided to volunteer one day a week at the canteen and over a few weeks, I read all the labels of the processed foods. I found that there were foods my child could safely eat. Because the canteen used a paper bag early order system, I let Victor have canteen food once a week, so he could be like other children and have something different.

Here is a sample of foods that he ate for breakfast, morning tea, lunch, afternoon tea and dinner.

BREAKFAST
Sanitarium Up & Go's
Weet Bix
Vita Brits
Fruity Bites
Sultana Bran
Cheerios
Toast with Butter & Vegemite, Honey, Cheesybite or Easy Spreading Cheese
Milk
Nesquik, Milo, Malted Milk
Plain Popcorn

MORNING & AFTERNOON TEAS

Fruit - Oranges, Apples, Bananas, Strawberries, Seedless Grapes
'LCM Yoghurt Splits' Bars - Vanilla, Chocolate
'Nutri-Grain' Bars
Tubs of fruit - peaches & two fruits
Fruits and Jelly
Tiny Teddies
Arnott's Shapes
Plain Popcorn
Fruity Bites
Sultanas
Tubes/ Tubs of Yoghurt/ Probiotics
Cheese sticks
Crackers and cheese dip
Potato chips, Twisties, French Fries occasionally for treats
Oreo chocolate-coated wafers
Fruit/ plain muffins
Sanitarium Up & Go's
Frozen fruit juice poppas
Purified bottled water

LUNCH

Cheese & Bacon Rolls
Vegemite, Honey, Cheesybite sandwiches
Ham sandwich
Cheese sandwich

CANTEEN LUNCH

Pizza Roundas
Ham & Pineapple Pizza
Hot Dogs with tomato sauce
Sausage Rolls
Frozen Yogurt
Milk drinks
Flavoured Mineral Water
N.B. **Salad sandwiches are great. Unfortunately, my child wouldn't eat salad. He was more a 'meat and potatoes' young man. (He still is.)

DINNERS

Store bought Barbecue Chicken
Chicken Nuggets
Lamb chops
Home-made rissoles
Poached eggs
Mashed, steamed, roasted potato
Steamed carrot, broccoli, corn
Frozen mixed vegetables
Herb/ garlic bread (without sesame seeds on top)

TAKEAWAYS/ TAKEOUTS

Chicken Nuggets and Chips/ Fries/ Wedges or Sliced Apple
Crumbed Fish and Chips/ Fries or Wedges
Ham & Pineapple Pizza
Sausage rolls & Meat pies
Hot dogs
Cheesy toast fingers & Raisin toast
BBQ chicken on fresh bread rolls (without sesame seeds on top)
Pancakes and ice-cream
Boysenberry, Mint or Strawberry drumsticks (without nuts on top)

N.B. * * Always check the cooking oil that the takeaway/ takeout family restaurant or shop uses to deep fry.

6. SUPPLEMENTS

'For the body to function in a healthy state for the term of a lifetime, vitamins and minerals, whether found naturally in foods or man-made are essential part of the diet.'

Along with providing Victor with nutritious food to help his body grow and stay well, I bought a good child's vitamin & mineral supplement and gave him and his brother one each day upon waking. By putting a supplement in their mouth, this helped both of them to wake up for school, but more importantly, supported their immune systems.

As a bonus, I found my children stopped getting colds one after another. I also believe multi-vitamins supported Victor's developing body, especially when he wasn't eating much food.

Vegebuddies (available at the Pharmacy or Health Food Store) were also excellent when Victor refused to eat two pieces of fruit and five vegetables every day. Vegebuddies contained nine different fruits and vegetables. (Victor only needed four per day. When he grew older, I increased it to six a day. He still gladly has them some days when he flatly refuses to eat fruit and vegetables.)

I found supplements helped immensely to relax the focus on food. Focusing on food was natural with a food allergy, but being obsessed about it, caused undue stress. If Victor was getting the foods from the five food groups over a week period with a supplement each day, I believed that he was healthy and normal. And he was. The same applied to Freddie.

7. NATURAL MEDICINE

'Natural Medicine has been used for eons by many cultures with little or no side effects.'

I found visits to my naturopath, homeopath and chiropractor were crucial in kick-starting my child's healing journey.

The naturopath was able to give me reassurance, as well as, nutritional and herbal supplements to help me stay well as my child's carer. They helped me cope with the high volumes of physical, emotional, mental and spiritual demands ahead.

The homeopath tested Victor for allergies. It was found that he was allergic to many foods - sugar, gluten, eggs, milk, red meat, nuts, as well as, dust mites and cat fur.

Everything my child was eating, our cat and the dust that was ever present in the house, in the air and at school was making my child sick.
I was devastated. Was I a bad mother? Why was this happening to my child?

But it wasn't only happening to my child. It was happening globally, to other people's children. Some say 20 per cent of the world's population.

I wasn't about to get rid of our beloved cat, Elle - a Persian/ Mogi cross. I only had the time and inclination to vacuum the house once a week. Dusting only happened twice a year!

Besides, I'd read that it was better for the child suffering the allergies, to be exposed to little bits of the allergens every now and then, to build up a tolerance to them, as they grew up.

Children often grew out of things - clothes, shoes, hats, why not allergies.

The Homeopath gave me some 'drops of wisps' of all the allergens to give my child over a period of time. I increased the number of drops daily to a peak level, and then decreased them over the course of a month, as instructed.

I then had to substitute all of the other food allergies: sugar with honey or the herb, Stevia; gluten (wheat-based products) with rice and corn-based products; eggs with powdered egg substitute; dairy milk with lactose-free, goat or rice milk; and red meat with chicken and fish.

This regime gave an effective detoxification of my child's body and took a heavy burden off his immune system.

The homeopathic drops gave my child's body a gentle way of reintroducing the allergens, including nuts.

After the month of detoxification and building up resilience in his body, I was able to slowly re-introduce those foods, one at a time, over several weeks.

During Spring, I had the cat shaved once a year. This reduced the amount of fur being shed in the house, but it was also helped Elle who was aging and feeling the Summer heat more. The cat and my child were arch-enemies. The only time they would come near each other, was when Victor was asleep and Elle would sleep at the end of his bed. I felt this was a gentle way of my child being exposed to cat fur, without patting her.

After a few months, I summoned up the courage to buy some Brazil nuts. I scraped a tiny amount of the nut and gave it to my child every day, until I lost my nerve, or Victor started to feel a bit sick in the stomach. I didn't tell him what it was, so that fear wouldn't be a factor, if any reaction was to occur.

Every six months, I gave a course of the drops until the drops ran out. I did the nut scrapings once a year for two years. (I've put this into the action plan earlier than I actually did it. I waited three months for an appointment with an Allergy Specialist first which was sheer agony.)

I also took my child to the Chiropractor regularly to make sure his skeletal system was aligned. This would help strengthen his immune system and keep his organs and cells functioning at optimum wellness.

One of our neighbours had an outdoor aviary in the backyard which was close to our bathroom window. As my child always felt ill after having a bath, I checked the birdseed the Cockatiels were eating at the supermarket. I found that it contained peanut and sesame seeds.

I decided then to close all the windows on that side of the house and asked everyone to keep them closed. As a result, my child didn't feel sick after having a bath anymore. (If you have caged birds, remember to check what's in their food.) I also checked dog, fish and cat food labels, but it is wise to check all foods for the pets in your family.

A few years later, the neighbours moved and took their aviary with them. We were then able to open the windows on that side of the house. I felt that it wasn't right to ask the neighbours to get rid of their beloved pets. Just as I knew I couldn't get rid of my beloved Elle. I'd found a practical way to close off the allergen. My child still played in the backyard. He wasn't affected by the birdseed there. It was only in the small enclosed area of the bathroom, when the doors were closed and the window left open during the day. When the room dried out after morning showers, the concentration of the allergen had intensified.

I'd like to thank my wonderful Naturopath, Robyn Ehmen (nee Miller), my Homeopath, Carol Schafer and Chiropractor/ Acupuncturist/ Naturopath, Dr Timothy Dunn, for all their wisdom and magnificent health care for my child and my whole family over many, many years.

I am eternally grateful to you all.

8. THE WHOLE SUPERMARKET THING

'The Supermarket is a library which proves hours of informative reading.'

Initially, every time I ventured out to the supermarket, I allowed two hours to do the grocery shopping. I had my husband, trusted friend or relative mind my children, while I focused on the task of reading labels and making lists of nut-free foods and foods that may contain traces of nuts.

N.B. ** My lists in the APPENDIX may help you as a starting point. (Do this several times until you have enough foods to provide a balanced and varied diet. One of which the whole family can eat.)

Making twenty-one different meals each week plus snacks was a logistical nightmare, especially when my husband and I were both working outside the home, on top of housekeeping and/ or yard work at home.

I still bought foods that my child couldn't eat because other family members enjoyed them. My husband has had a peanut butter sandwich every day of his working life and still does. I have always eaten mixed nuts every day. My son, Freddie often eats muesli bars containing nuts for lunch and snacks.

On one of my fact-finding trips, I checked out toiletries and cleaning products. I found natural cleaning products to be nut-free. Many shampoos, soaps, hair-gels, hair dyes, make-up, etc., contain nut oil, especially almond. **Check everything you normally use for facial cleansers, toners, moisturisers, sunscreen and insect repellent, for your own peace of mind.

N.B. ** (Kissing your child with foundation or lipstick containing nut oil may cause a reaction in your child.)

Personally I have foregone the use of make-up, except on special occasions, but I use a nut-free lipstick and moisturiser every day.

The same goes for men. Check shaving creams, gels, soaps, deodorants and aftershaves. My husband only uses an all-in-one shampoo and conditioner, plain oatmeal and degreasing soaps, so there are no problems there.

N.B. ** Remember to ask the hairdresser, what is in the products they are using in the salon. It is better to ask if they contain any nut oil, than to have your child go through an anaphylactic reaction. (Almond Oil is a common ingredient.)

I've always checked out new food products on the shelves. Often they are advertised and children want to try them. It may add more variety to their diet. Recently, to my child's delight, I found a nut-free muesli bar. Rice bubble bars can get very boring.

9. NOTIFICATION

'Food Companies appreciate feedback to better serve the public.'

I wrote to the maker of the product to which Victor had had a reaction immediately, notifying them that my child had had a reaction to their Brazil Nut Chocolate.

I also asked where the Brazil nuts came from and if there was any kind of coating/ preservative on them.

As it happened, several people had had a reaction to their Brazil Nut Chocolate and it was immediately removed from the supermarket shelves. I haven't seen it there since!

Unfortunately, I threw away the rest of the chocolate. Perhaps, if I had kept it, it may have been able to be analysed.

A few months later, I gave my child a little piece of that company's plain chocolate. There was no reaction, so I believed that he wasn't allergic to the chocolate. He continues to eat plain chocolate today.

N.B. ** It is not the company's fault that my child had had a reaction to their product so I did not blame them. It was better to use my energies and resources in caring for and healing my child from anaphylactic reactions.

10. ENVIRONMENTAL FACTORS

'There are many things we can control to prevent an anaphylactic reaction but there are also many we can't.'

It was important that I identified any environmental factors which may have had a causal link to the anaphylactic reaction, through suppression of the immune system.

As mentioned earlier, I observed what things may be affecting my child. For example: Birdseed, plants, grass, dust, mites & fleas, mosquitoes, bees & wasps, pollens, pollution, yard fertilisers and chemicals for weed control, pets, etc.

Victor, when bitten by a mosquito, would have a severe reaction. The sight of the bitten area would blow up to the size of a golf ball. If a mosquito bit him on the throat, I knew his windpipe would be cut off. When my naturopath found Victor had low amounts of Thiamine (part of the vitamin B complex) in his system, increasing his Thiamine levels reduced the severity of the reaction. (Now that vitamin B complex is included in Victor's daily supplement, he is mosquito bite reaction free.)

Some children have an anaphylactic reaction if the allergen is airborne. At school, if someone near them is eating a peanut butter or Nutella (a chocolate spread which contains hazelnuts) sandwich or a nut-based muesli bar, a reaction would occur. For this reason, nut spreads and products are banned in many schools and kindergartens.

I know some parents who have chosen to home school their children for this reason, but it may have repercussions to their wellbeing. This is especially so, if they are too afraid to allow them to do any activity in the community.

I also know some parents who sit outside their child's school all day, paralysed with fear.

The 'Prayer of Serenity' is wise to follow here: God grant me the courage to accept the things we cannot change; to change the things we can; and to gain the wisdom to know the difference.

N.B.**At this point, it is appropriate to mention for those religious children taking Communion in churches that they will require a separate little cup of wine. Many of the ladies who attend church wear foundation and lipstick. Their make-up may contain nut oil. Parishioners may also have eaten something containing nuts for breakfast and traces of nuts may still be in their mouths. (In this day and age, all drinking wine from the one cup is downright dangerous, something akin to Russian roulette!)

11. PREVENTION, PREVENTION, PREVENTION

'When someone is aware that something is bad for their health, it is their choice to abide by the warning for their own well-being.'

Education is important to consistently prevent an anaphylactic reaction to nuts. CPR doesn't work. Only giving an adrenaline shot in the form of an Epi-Pen Junior/ Epi-Pen within the first couple of minutes of the body's cellular system shutting down, gives a child with this life-threatening condition, any chance of survival.

Prevention must occur long before an anaphylactic reaction. Victor had already required two adrenaline shots to initially survive. The nurse had also forewarned me that this form of First Aid may or may not work next time.

Within the three months' time span waiting to attend the Allergist's Appointment, Victor came to me after taking a bath. He said that he couldn't breathe. He was terrified and was working himself up into a state fuelled by anxiety and fear.

Though I felt sheer panic course through my veins, for some reason, my years of First Aid training kicked in. Firstly, I looked at Victor from head to toe for any signs and symptoms of an allergic reaction. His face was blotchy and his breathing was short and shallow with a little wheeze.

His face hadn't puffed up like before and there was no red circle on his throat. He also hadn't eaten anything containing nuts. Was there something in the bathroom making him sick? Had someone accidentally opened the window? Was there a toiletry that I hadn't checked that contained nut oil?

Immediately, I rang the paramedics and had the Epi-Pen Junior nearby. I chose not to give him the adrenaline shot. He was still breathing by himself.

Remaining calm, I stayed with him and hummed a lullaby, while stroking down his arms.

By the time the paramedics arrived, Victor was breathing much better. The paramedics examined him and decided to transport him to hospital, as per their policies and procedures. They also didn't feel the need to give him an adrenaline shot.

Freddie came with me, as Adam was still at work. When we arrived at the local hospital, Victor was taken straight into a room set up for children.

A nurse put Victor on a nebuliser to assist his breathing and to open his airway while we waited for a doctor to examine him. There were children's books there, so I read to both my children.

We waited an hour until a very busy doctor came. Though Victor was breathing normally, the doctor ordered a shot of Phenergan (anti-histamine) as per procedure. We waited another twenty minutes, until the doctor announced that we could go home.

I called Adam to pick us up from the hospital. It was then reality hit and he believed that Victor had some sort of mysterious condition. His knee-jerk reaction was to buy me my first mobile/ cell phone. It came in handy a lot of times, none of which, thankfully, was to ring the paramedics after an anaphylactic reaction.

What I did realise from the experience, however, was that fear and anxiety played a huge part in the body's speed and intensity of the reaction. I also wondered if the more adrenaline and anti-histamine shots my child had, would he eventually become immune to it, so it wouldn't work at all.
I decided then and there that prevention was the best cure for anaphylactic reactions.

I also had to learn to distinguish the difference in signs and symptoms between anxiety, asthma and chest colds. Victor has never had asthma, but having had an anxiety attack once, I believed anxiety was mimicking asthma symptoms, especially difficulty in breathing.

Being diligent, I informed everyone in contact with Victor about his condition and taught him to read labels.

These were the keys to prevention.

Victor was in a multi-age class with two teachers and sixty children. One day, both his teachers were away. One of the relief/ supply teachers gave him a chocolate bar, as a reward for working well in class.
Before eating it, he read the label as I had taught him to do before putting anything unfamiliar in his mouth. On the bottom of the label, it stated that the product may contain traces of nuts. He showed the teacher, and then told her that he couldn't have it because he was allergic to nuts.

The supply teacher was unaware of his allergy. She was devastated that she could have killed him. That prompted me to inform Administration that all supply/ relief teachers needed to be aware of children with medical conditions, in the classroom that they were teaching.

Other children and adults give treats often, so in that case and so many others, it was invaluable for my child to identify the words that could prevent him from having a reaction. (Even if children are really young, they may be able to understand, that if there are any words in bold type that stand out, they are not to eat it, until they learn to read and/ or to ask an adult about what the label says.

Prevention works. It helps your child live a normal, healthy life.

12. DEALING WITH FEAR AND ANXIETY

'Fear is the mind telling the body to fight or runaway when feeling threatened by real or imaginary demons.'

By remaining calm and educating Victor and the rest of the family as well, my child has never had another anaphylactic reaction. Even during Winter, when he'd caught heavy, chest colds and he'd felt that he couldn't breathe, by remaining calm and understanding that it wasn't an anaphylactic reaction to nuts, he always healed quickly and responded well with over-the-counter medicine obtained at a Pharmacy.

Some techniques that help with learning to remain calm are:
- Meditation
- Yoga
- Prayer
- Giving Emergency Flower Essence Drops

I have practiced and used them all. They also helped me to learn to stay in the moment and to be grateful for each and every one.

I don't own Victor. He was a gift to my husband and I and our family. A beautiful blessing.

13. FACING DEATH

'Death, like taxes, is inevitable, as long as you live long enough to pay them.'

Early on, I'd accepted that Victor could die any tick of the clock.

My mother gave birth to still-born twin girls at eight and half months. Those babies, sadly taken by flu virus in-uteri, didn't get to the chance to take even a single breath. I can only imagine the pain and grief that my mother went through. I was only a year old at the time.

My great aunt, Doris lived until one hundred and three. Several of her children died in their sixties. Though they lived full lives, the pain and grief of losing your child was still the same - immense.

Victor was nine when he told me that he'd had his first dream. He dreamt that he'd flown to Townsville by aeroplane.

There were two things miraculous about this dream. Firstly, he didn't know Townsville existed (a North Queensland tropical city in Australia). Secondly, he was terrified of flying after watching a television show on aeroplane crashes.

Shortly after the dream, my husband and I received an invitation to attend my cousin, Lee's eldest daughter's wedding. It was to take place in the Outback of Northern Queensland, nine hours' drive from Townsville.

My husband didn't want to go, as he had neither met the bride nor groom. I knew Coral, the bride, when she was young and had once taken her on her first camel ride. One of my close aunts, Heather was now living in the Outback, being cared for by her children, as she battled breast cancer for the second time. I wanted to see her one last time and told my husband that I really needed to go. I also told him about Victor's dream and felt that he also needed to attend the wedding.

Adam thought I was crazy, taking a boy with a nut allergy, where there was no hospital, doctors or communications. It was very risky but somehow, I knew that if Victor faced death, that he would have the courage to live a full life. He would believe that "anything is possible you set your mind to, for the good of all". It was something I often said to my boys, which meant something akin to "the sky's the limit!"

My cousin, Kenny and his wife, Marie were supposed to share a hire car with us from Townsville Airport. Kenny, who had driven into the Outback before, was supposed to drive.

Alas, a couple of days prior to departure, Kenny landed in hospital with a mysterious, life-threatening infection in his throat. After two operations, they'd managed to save him, but he wasn't strong enough to make the journey.

Henceforth, Victor and I set off alone. With no experience driving in the Outback, I soon realised, I was way out of my depth. Wildlife, road trains and endless dirt and bitumen roads that alternated every couple of kilometres/ miles between a single and a double road were nerve-wracking enough. However, when night time fell and we were shrouded in darkness with only time and distance our guides, it was even more terrifying and less controllable, I suddenly realised, than having a nut allergy.

We stopped at a town called, Charter's Towers, as I'd been told there was a supermarket there. Unsure of what food would be available at our destination, Mount Surprise, I purchased meat, frozen vegetables, milk, cereal, water, bread, butter, Vegemite and a couple of pieces of fruit. I used the frozen vegetables, as the ice pack in the cooler bag, to keep things cool, as my ice pack had already thawed in the immense, tropical, dry heat.

By stopping in Charter's Towers, it added four hours to the journey. Though it doesn't sound much extra, for a mother used to local driving to drop the children at school and to do the shopping at the Mall, I was so far out of my comfort zone; I may as well have been on a rocket to Mars!

It was 7:30 p.m. by the time we reached the last Roadhouse before Mount Surprise. It was pitch-black and we were badly in need of fuel.
The latest model sedan I'd hired was air-conditioned, reliable and beautiful to drive, but it only took E10 fuel. The Roadhouse only had diesel and regular petrol at the bowsers.

After the kind-hearted, elderly lady had thankfully provided Victor with a nut-free dinner, I asked her what would happen if the car broke down, because it wasn't the right fuel.

She replied in a foreboding voice, 'It's a long, lonely road.'

A shiver of fear coursed down my spine and visions of old Australian movies, where people had broken down in the Outback and had perished or been murdered, reeled through my tired, overwrought brain.

We were already an hour and a half overdue. No one came looking for us. There was no way of contacting them even though the efficient, young lady at the car hire counter had assured me that my mobile/ cell phone would work in the Outback. It didn't.

We continued on, tired and apprehensive. A large white owl tumbled into the windscreen. Terror had planted my foot heavily on the accelerator. I was doing way over a hundred kilometres per hour/ sixty miles per hour. The fastest I'd ever driven. It took all my strength to keep control of the car and bring it to a halt.
My heart pumping, I started again. I had learnt earlier on in the day that the biggest vehicle on the road had right of way. Only one smaller car had

pulled to the side of the road to let us pass. Most people drove utilities/ pick-ups, four wheel drives or trucks. Sensible cars for driving in the Outback. If only I'd thought to hire a four wheel drive!

When we'd spotted two large globes coming towards us, I'd guessed it was a road train, but there was no way of telling how far away it was or how fast it was travelling.

My stomach churned. By instinct alone, I pulled the car up as fast as I could and steered to the side of the road as far as I dared with only the headlights for vision.

Shortly after, the road train rumbled past at breakneck speed. We breathed in and squeezed our eyes shut tight as if we were about to die. The whole car shuddered as the rig with six trailers snaking behind hissed by.

After surviving that ordeal, we exhaled heavily. We then started taking turns of what we were grateful for in our lives. It had a calming and healing effect on both of us. Victor was exhausted and I told him it was alright for him to go to sleep.

After he'd nodded off, I turned up the air-conditioning and the CD player and planted my foot to the floor once more. Without a second of regret, I knew Victor and I had shared an epiphany about life and the importance of enjoying each and every moment of our lives. Life was about the journey, not the destination.

Ninety minutes later, I spotted a tiny sign, but I couldn't make out what it said as I was travelling too fast. It took a hundred or so metres/ one hundred and ten yards to pull the car up and somehow manoeuvre it around on the narrow road.

Sure enough, the sign said Mount Surprise and pointed down an even narrower side road. Another ninety minutes later, dog-tired, but elated that I had endured such an arduous drive at the wheel; I pulled the car into the Jo and Joe's Caravan Park at Mount Surprise. It was pitch-black. At ten o'clock at night, all were asleep.

Scared of creepy crawlies and no way of knowing if there were any poisonous or dangerous wildlife around, I drove straight up to what-I-thought-to-be the owner's house and shone the headlights into the front window.

Moments later, Victor and I were settled into a beautiful cabin with all the mod-cons. Mount Surprise was truly full of surprises.
After a much-needed rest, the next morning, Victor went for a swim in the pool, while I became acquainted with the neighbours, who just happened to be the priest, who was performing the wedding nuptials and his wife.

Somehow it was comforting to know if Victor needed his last rites, there was a clergyman there to perform it.

One by one, we met many of our relatives who were staying in the Caravan Park. The entire town's people were invited to the wedding and a bus was provided to carry us further into the belly of a cattle station another ninety minute drive into the heart of the Outback.

After the marriage ceremony, drinks were provided at the pub on the property. Then it was on to the reception. Held at a race track, the only facilities were a toilet block, which housed two toilets labelled "Cows" and "Bulls." The hand washing water was underground bore water.

With no fresh water or anything non-alcoholic for Victor to drink, our next survival test was before us.

Parched by the dusty, dry, searing heat of the Outback, Victor inevitably asked me for something to quench his thirst. As the sun set a vivid orange over an endless barren landscape, I set about visiting every ice box set around the grounds. All were filled with either beer or champagne. Hidden behind a shed, I struck gold in the form of cans of lemonade/ soda. It was possibly a private ice box, but with over two hundred people in attendance, I had no way of asking to whom it belonged. In sheer desperation, I did something I never thought I would ever do. I took a can and gave it to Victor.

I'd like to thank the person who thought to bring something for the children to drink. They were truly a lifesaver that night!

When it came time for the wedding dinner, I talked with the caterers who had cooked and prepared the food in a town eight hours away. They assured me that they'd taken the utmost care with the ingredients. The oil and some salads were the most obvious to contain nuts.

After the wedding party had gathered their food, I was allowed to prepare a plate for Victor. This gave minimal chance of cross-contamination of food. Not one to eat salads made it infinitely easier.

The next day we relaxed by taking in the local tourist attraction, the spectacular Undullah Lava Caves. There we played pool before heading back to the Caravan Park for a game of nine-hole mini-golf. Victor enjoyed himself immensely.

Though my cousin, Lee had asked me to visit her at her home, another two hours' drive away; I knew I'd reached my limit of stress. I couldn't drive any further into the Outback. My nerves were shot. I still had to summon the courage to drive back to Townsville the next day – a five hour shortcut through the unknown mountain terrain.

The food I had bought with me looked a little dubious, as it had been out of refrigeration for nine hours. Not knowing that the Caravan Park owners did stock a variety of food for sale, I believed I had no choice, but to cook up the meat and vegetables and hope that we didn't get food poisoning. Luckily, we didn't.

The journey was a turning point in our lives. We realised that many things could kill a person in the blink of an eye. If death was meant to be, then it was meant to be.

Victor and I were grateful for everything in our lives so far and we thanked the occurrence of the nut allergy to draw our attention to it.

Accepting death, as part of life, was the commencement of Victor being able to trust enough in life to heal himself.

The Outback wedding was magnificent and very unique. Coral and her bridesmaids (three of them her sisters - Lorna, Shelley and Kerrin)looked stunning in their long wedding couture dresses against the backdrop of the Einsleigh River - a long ribbon of water which cut a striking path through a centuries old lava flow of now dark, basalt rock. The groom, Noel and his groomsmen in their country attire and ten-gallon hats, sipped on tinnies (cans of beer) grabbed from an ice box on the back of a utility truck, while waiting for the bridal party to descend a carpeted path, down a slippery embankment. Line dancing, a live country band and a wedding cake, shaped in a country coach drawn by six chestnut horses, complete with beer kegs on the back, all made for unforgettable memories.

To see my relatives again, especially Aunt Heather one last time before her passing, gave me the utmost understanding and respect of people who make their lives in the harsh and yet majestic environment called, The Outback.

14. NORMAL HEALTHY LIVING

'Life isn't black and white. There are many shades of colour.'

Something changed in Victor on that trip. He became more confident that he could take care of himself under any circumstance. He'd overcome his fear of flying and the following year was able to join his class on a trip to the Snowy Mountains, which included return plane trips from Brisbane to Sydney.

Victor embraced life. He went to school, participated in school musicals, played musical instruments, entered science competitions, went on school camps, participated in sporting teams (soccer & cricket), and went to birthday parties, fetes, cinemas, laser skirmishes and even sleep-overs.

I was very grateful to my friends who were willing to care for Victor, as their own, on sleep-overs. Though they were concerned that Victor might die under their watch, I still pushed through those fears with practical wisdom and courage. They worked out that if they made home-cooked food without nuts/ nut oil; there wouldn't be a chance of an allergic reaction. They took the time to learn how to use the Epi-Pen Junior/ Epi-Pen and kept it in a handy place.

Thank you to Wendy & Kevin, Jane & John, Susan & Edward, Anna & Douglas, Lisa & Malcolm, and Jennifer & Bradley. I'd also like to thank Victor's Nan for making lots of home-made, nut-free birthday cakes and goodies over the years; and his Godmother, Margeaux and his Uncle Luke for minding, caring and feeding him. Uncle Luke also spent many, many hours with Victor in the backyard developing his all-round cricket skills. He also gave me lots of support and practical advice.

The day of my Uncle Henry's funeral was the day of Victor's long-awaited Allergist Appointment - an appointment that took three months to obtain. Once I went to the appointment, I had imagined that the Allergist would hold the key to miraculously healing him and all our worries would be over.

Uncle Henry had said before he'd died, that *he'd more to do in life, that he wasn't ready to die.*

I didn't want Victor to feel that way. The world was his oyster and he had plenty of time to fulfil his bucket list at the ripe old age of eight.

Excited by the prospect of answers, we arrived at the hospital where the Allergist's room was situated.

To our disappointment, according to the Allergist, there was no concrete reason for a nut allergy to occur out of the blue. I'd read theories about not letting little ones play in the dirt to build up their immune system; about mothers-to-be eating nuts while pregnant; about preservatives; genetically-modified foods and pollution; but nothing was set in stone.

Victor was given an allergy prick test on the inside of his forearm. Each prick had a little of common allergen substances - peanuts, almonds, dairy milk, eggs, soybeans, gluten, wheat and Brazil nuts.

After waiting the allotted time, the Allergist pronounced that Victor was allergic to all of them to varying degrees, the most reactive being the nut protein. He was allergic to all nuts and not allowed any in his diet.

The Allergist then said to bring him back for another test in three months or when he turned eighteen. Still shocked by his diagnosis, I thought this was a bizarre thing to say.

Did I bring him back in three months due to fear, or to see if the allergies were the same or better or worse? Why bring him back at eighteen? Was it possible to outgrow an anaphylactic reaction to nuts? I hadn't read anywhere that it was possible. There was some talk of giving a series of injections of the allergens over a period of time. Maybe at eighteen, as an adult, Victor could choose to do this.

Was it possible to change, lessen or abolish the reaction entirely? There was some evidence on reputable websites that by introducing little bits of the allergen into the child's diet, they might not react so severely to it.

In a state of mental numbness, I could only ask the Allergist, 'He's eating everything you say he's allergic to. What do I feed him?'
After a pause, his answer was, 'Chicken Balls.'

I'm sure the look on my face was sheer astonishment. How did he expect a child or anyone for that matter to eat Chicken Balls (which Victor had never eaten before) for breakfast, lunch and dinner?

Seeing the helplessness and compassion in the Allergist's eyes, I thanked him. The unspoken words were, 'Take him home, and love him until death comes.'

When I arrived outside, the sun beat on my face. I gripped Victor's hand and walked him across the road. Hungry, we had lunch at a popular fast food restaurant and I vowed then and there that I would find a way to heal Victor one hundred per cent.

Twenty percent of all children worldwide have a nut allergy, there had to be a way to help every single one of them overcome this condition. Suddenly, I knew this was my mission in life. What I was born to do.

We headed back to my Uncle Henry's wake and celebrated his life with his family and relatives. I also asked the elder women of the family if they had a recipe for chicken balls - that was suitable for Victor to eat given all his newfound allergies - and most importantly, chicken balls he would eat, given that he was such a fussy eater!

What we came up with was this:

45

Victor's Chicken Ball Recipe

Ingredients

500g fresh chicken mince
20g substitute egg powder & purified water
Salt & paprika
Rice flour
Olive oil

Method

1. Mix chicken mince, egg substitute and a little salt & paprika for seasoning in a bowl.
2. Roll a teaspoon of the chicken mixture into little balls and then roll them in the rice flour.
3. Fry all the balls in a little olive oil.
4. Drain and cool on paper towels.
5. Wrap the balls in packs of three or four in plastic wrap for individual meals.
6. Place in freezer.

By having these little easy to reheat morsels of protein, it made cooking family dinners less taxing. By putting steamed vegetables and rice, rice pasta or herb bread with meat and a sauce for the rest of the family, it was simple to make a square meal for Victor.

A trip to the Health Food Shop provided him with a range of rice cereals, corn cakes, gluten-free biscuits & plain potato chips. But it was mainly sticking to whole foods that gave Victor a healthy, balanced diet.

I took him to the Naturopath/ Homeopath and we started again to detox his body of all the toxins causing the allergies and putting pressure on his immune system.

In effect, anaphylactic nut allergies are a form of A.I.D.S. - Auto-Immune Dis-ease Syndrome.

To me, that meant that many things were causing Victor to shut his life down.

From my observations and life experience, Louise L. Hay's wisdom seemed feasible in understanding the psychological cause of Victor attracting this affliction into his life.

A.I.D.S. seems to be caused by a thought pattern where someone is not happy with who they are. They believe that they aren't good enough to be here. (Hay, 1984)

Could Victor have an inferiority complex because he'd had delayed speech? Was he being ridiculed or bullied at school because of it? Was living in his older brother's high achieving shadow affecting his self-esteem?

46

It was certainly possible.

I also looked at the psychological cause of chronic dis-eases which was caused by stubborn thoughts of not wanting to change and not wanting to or feeling safe about moving forward in life. (Hay, 1984)

Victor would often come out with negative sayings like: 'He'd had a bad day. The day was bad, bad, bad. It just kept getting worse.' It was like he was dialling into and spiralling into a vortex of negativity and darkness.

To get him out of this negativity, I would talk to him about the good or positive things that happened to me that day and asked him to find something good that happened to him and focus on that.

On a regular basis, I also said to him affirmations to change his thought patterns.

Victor was a Capricorn, born in the Year of the Ox. He was a very stubborn character and would dig his heels in so hard, the only way I found to get him to move was through humour.

Victor also had a Jim Carrey-type sense of humour for the absurd. He liked watching Weird Al Yanovich's parodies of famous songs on You Tube; cartoons on the television like The Simpsons, American Dad, South Park, The Cleveland Show, Futurama and The Big Bang Theory. He also liked Mythbusters, Good News Week, Spicks'n'Specks and Top Gear. All were very funny shows. Victor would often do his own parodies on songs and make up funny lyrics to his own melodies.

While we ate dinner, I would play relaxation music and taking a family tradition from the movie, "The Deep End of the Ocean" ask the family to talk about their high and low time of each day. This helped Victor see that there was balance in every day. No day was totally bad or totally good.

I also brought him to see a showing of the movie, "The Secret" by Rhonda Byrne. Afterwards, he stood up and danced around happily saying that it all made sense to him and that he was going to be wealthy and rich in spirit.

Understanding the power of being grateful for everything in life helped him to happily embrace the present and his future with a certainty that everything would be safe, well and good.

Those dug-in goat heels were starting to shift forward and move freely into his future.

I looked at his seven year life cycles. (Some use nine year cycles.) Victor had struggled through his first seven physical years adjusting to life on Earth. Now he was dealing with understanding human emotions.

About this time, I had the opportunity to do a parenting course mainly to do with communicating better with my husband and children. I learnt by role modelling positive, Win-Win conversations with my husband, that my children would gain a better insight into using their emotional intelligence, thinking destructive thoughts before opening their mouth.

By communicating well, my children learnt that their thoughts and feelings were real and important and that they could express them in a positive way, instead of taking energy in the form of happiness from others.

I realised then and there that to heal Victor, I had to treat the whole person on physical, emotional, mental and spiritual levels.

15. ACTIVITIES IN THE COMMUNITY

'As developmental milestones occurred, I treated the boys exactly the same.'

Ever since my children could walk, I would take them for short treks in the forest a couple of afternoons a week to get their energy out and to ensure a good night's sleep.

In the local forest, there were three treks of varying lengths - 1 kilometre/ 0.62 miles, 8 kilometres/ 4.97 miles and 14 kilometres/ 8.7 miles. We did the 1 kilometre/ 0.62 mile tree-identifying trek for many years. When they had grown and Victor had the nut allergy, we attempted the 8 kilometre/ 4.97 mile trek successfully. Two years later, we walked all day to complete the final and most enduring 14 kilometre/ 8.7 mile trek.

After that, we hiked in State Forests and scaled mountains. Stamina, persistence and tenacity were the life lessons to be learnt there.
Bike riding through bike parks were also something we did regularly as a family.

For years, I'd informed Freddie, my eldest son that he wasn't allowed by law to ride on his own, until he turned ten. When he was about ten and a half, he informed me that he was going for a ride around the neighbourhood. I could see determination in his eyes. He was ready for adventure, to spread his wings of independence. I replied, 'I'll get my camera.'

The boys knew I documented everything in photographs, so he kindly waited until I fetched my camera and snapped off a photograph of his first solo bike ride.

Being second born, as soon as Victor turned ten, he announced that he too was off to explore the neighbourhood on his bike. Again, I said, 'Wait until I get my camera.'

Like a fledgling bird, he too needed to take his first flight of independence.

Later, much later, the boys confessed to riding through four or five suburbs on some of their rides. Victor rode the furthest to the next city. Adam was horrified, concerned for his safety, as Victor hadn't told anyone where he was going or slipped his Epi-Pen Junior into his backpack.

I, on the other hand, congratulated him on his willingness to get out in the world, though I did remind him the next day to let someone know where he was going. Riding one's own bicycle was not a high risk for having an anaphylactic reaction.

I also reminded Adam that he was an adventurer as a child. He'd even joined a trailblazer's club in his late teens. My siblings and I had also regularly explored the neighbourhood. It was a normal thing to do in childhood.

Victor was a member of a soccer team at the later named Loganholme Lightning Football Club. He had been with them since Under 6's. I was the team's manager and worked with several dedicated, excellent coaches passionate for the game.

Over the years, the boys developed excellent team and individual ball skills. Often they won trophies at carnivals. Victor stayed with the team through the Rooball years and did a year in Divisional Football, before changing to Cricket.

Every year, he would attend the Club's Presentation Day. Thousands of parents and children would attend. There were rides and food, trophies and fireworks. Fantastic fun and a logistical nightmare for a child with a nut allergy.

In the middle of the field, I sat in a collapsible chair with the Epi-Pen Junior/ Epi-Pen in my handbag and read a book, while he had the time of his life.

From the age of nine, Victor had played Club, School Boy and District Cricket with the Beenleigh Cutters. His Loganholme Cobras Cricket Club had won two cricket training clinics with former Australian Wicket Keeper, Ian Healy. It was a very special, amazing experience for Victor and his team mates.

Victor gained many skills and much confidence in his abilities. His comedic skills also came in handy keeping the team entertained with his wry commentaries of each game.

A sporty kid, he picked up many friends during his childhood and only ended up in hospital twice during that time, both times with broken arms.

Out in the community, Victor proved that he could survive by his own wits. He was growing into a positive, confident, young man.
I had learned along the way that a prominent, local politician also had a nut allergy. He worked out at the gym, kept his body strong and healthy. A person in the public eye who attended many catered functions coped with his condition well with pre-planning and by being selective at the venue.

He was an inspiration to Victor that one could aspire to any form of employment. A nut allergy was not a major deterrent.

It also brought to my attention, that if Victor did become in the public eye, it was important to keep his allergy a secret. Mentally unstable members of the community could use nuts as a lethal weapon against him.

16. REWARDS AND RELAXATION

'The most important thing in life is health. Without good health, quality of life diminishes.'

Rewards bring joy and relaxation is needed to have breaks from stress and worry.

Worry was my constant companion. If the cells had no introduction of the nut protein, I fathomed that when Victor came in contact with it, the reaction would be severe.

On a positive note, I had also read that children had more chance of growing out of the nut allergy, if it was slowly reintroduced.

After detoxing Victor's body of all his allergens, I slowly reintroduced them all. I did this detoxification about once every six months. I also gave the homeopathic drops every six months with no adverse effects.

The only slight reaction Victor had during those first two years was to a processed quiche. He felt a little sick in the stomach, so I asked him to stop eating it. He soon felt better.

Each year, I would introduce new foods into his diet - some he liked and others he didn't. He started eating other home-made dinners on sleep-overs, which expanded his diet immensely.

Once a week, as a reward, I bought him a nut-free meal at one of the popular fast food restaurants. However, we stayed away from Chinese takeaway/ takeouts, due to so many of their menus containing nuts. I also felt it was too risky with their regular use of peanut and sesame oil.

The rest of the family loved Chinese food, so often I would make it at home with meat, rice and bottled ready-made sauces. By his own choice, Victor would eat the rice, chicken and vegetables without the sauce.

Barbecues and Sausage Sizzles were also another risky meal at school or other people's places. Often marinades and peanut satays were used on barbecue meats and therefore could be on the barbecue plate.

Recently, we've started having regular family barbecues at home using olive oil and cooking plain steak, rissoles, sausages and onion on the barbecue plate. Adam cooks, so it is a lovely reward for me.

Victor would often win class awards and sporting trophies. We put them on his bedroom walls and shelves respectively. This helped his self-worth and self-esteem immensely. With consistent praise, he learnt to believe in himself and a lot of his negativity about life ceased.

We started taking holidays. Each night, we would eat out. Commandeering the chef's help at cafes, restaurants and regular takeaway/ takeout places, we would easily find something Victor could eat. Staying in a resort-style hotel helped, so that we could store and make foods for the other meals of the day. It was a way to make great, relaxing memories.

Between the ages of nine and thirteen, I taught Victor how to make simple meals and snacks, so he could feed himself when hungry. Some of the food items were toast, grilled cheese on toast, poached eggs, canned spaghetti, pancakes, fruit and ice-cream, choc chip muffins and brownies.

By doing this, the pressure to feed him constantly reduced and he was enabled to care for himself.

I knew this was the key to him living independently as an adult.

17. BIRTHDAY PARTIES & SLEEP-OVERS

'Good memories are made from fun times with family and friends.'

When Victor's Nan was unable to make her fabulous novelty birthday cakes anymore for health reasons, we started having ice-cream cakes come Summer or Winter, morning or night. They were nut-free and easy to buy from the supermarket.

When Victor was invited to his friend's or classmates' birthday parties, I would buy him a nut-free meal at a popular fast food restaurant before he went, so that he wasn't hungry at the party. This reduced the risk of him eating party food, especially if he was unsure about it. It also reduced the pressure on the parents who hosted the parties. Victor was also content because he'd had a treat beforehand and his tummy was full.

Other things I would do include:
- Arriving early, if home-based parties, to help the parents prepare for the party.
- Asking the parents to remove all nuts and nut products from the party beforehand.
- Explaining First Aid - how to use the Epi-Pen Junior/ Epi-Pen and to call the paramedics, before calling me.
- Letting them know that First Aid may or may not work. I only asked them to give it a go.
- Suggesting that children have their names written on their disposable party cups with permanent marker to prevent cross-contamination.
- Picking up my child exactly on finishing time.
- Thanking the parents for inviting Victor to their child's party.
- Letting the parents know that it was okay for Victor to swim in their pool, if they were having a pool party.

When Victor turned nine, sleep-over parties started to become fashionable. Mostly, they would eat pizzas and play video games.

I am very grateful for those lovely friends and parents who were willing to take care of Victor. It gave Adam and I much needed respite. Again, I would always pick Victor up at the designated time next morning.

I also held reciprocated sleep-overs with their children. Some of those children had other medical/ psychological issues, so I also gave their parents much needed respite.

Now that Victor was a teenager, at fourteen, he would often stay all weekend at mates' places or they would spend time together moving from house to house to house for variety, depending on what technological/ swimming resources were available at each house. Sometimes, they'd hang out after school at the Mall; catch a movie at the cinema; go bowling or do indoor laser skirmish. Normal teenage fare.

18. EATING OUT

'Eating out is a normal and enjoyable part of family and social life.'

Picnics were easy. I would take all the food and drinks we would need. Finding food became an adventure, when we went out for a Sunday Drive to explore the surrounding environs. Wherever we stopped, I would consult with the chef/ cook and they would always do their utmost to give Victor a hearty meal.

Besides, the chain takeaway/ takeout fare, Victor ate sausage rolls, beef pies, pancakes and ice-cream, cheesy toast fingers, raisin toast, boysenberry drumsticks, hot dogs, BBQ chicken on fresh bread rolls (without sesame seeds on top), ham and pineapple pizzas and fish'n'chips. The cooking oil was the main ingredient that needed to be checked. Often oil would come in big drums and the chef would gladly read the ingredients. If it was blended oil from Asia, I usually stayed away from it, because peanut and sesame oils were often made in those factories. Plain canola, olive, vegetable and rice oils were all okay for Victor to eat. Buying plain rolls without sesame seeds on top was also a must.

Taking purified water, juice or soft drink/ soda and individual colour-coded cups for the family, also made outings joyful and effortless.

Taking lots of food and drinks to sporting carnivals was important for most parents; even more important for Victor.

Though Adam or I went to all of Victor's sporting/ musical events, it took some convincing for his coaches to train in the use of the Epi-Pen Junior. This was essential, for I, as team manager, was often elsewhere on the grounds sorting or fees and paperwork. If Victor had a bad reaction to something, then someone else needed to know what the First Aid procedures were.

I found all sporting clubs were happy to have Victor as a member. He had the opportunity to have fun and develop his athletic skills like any other sporty child.

At big events, where there were great crowds of people, such as: sporting arenas; theme parks; and the Exhibition, we employed the same methods to hunt down the foods, he could safely eat. On arrival, I would also notify the First Aid Officers, where we were seated.

19. TRAVEL AND HOLIDAYS

'Most people enjoy a break from everyday life.'

Travel and holidays are a part of everyday life. Most people want to explore their country, have holidays to the beach, on an island or in the countryside.

Victor has flown on an aeroplane several times, ridden on buses, trains, boats and ferries. He's been four-wheel driving, fishing, camping and hiking.

By being practical, being prepared and taking each moment as it comes, Victor has been on holiday, in many places in Australia.

I believe by applying the same principles, Victor could also travel overseas. Most people in the world I have found in my own travels before having children are compassionate and trustworthy. Communication and language are most important. There are Fast Food chains in almost every corner of the globe and supermarkets are good places to find everyday food. Open markets usually have a variety of whole foods. Victor would always find something he could eat and drink, if his life takes him overseas in the future.

What is important is the inspiration to experience all aspects of life, that he wants or needs, in his own given time.

Everything that happens to you is for a reason. It is part of the perfect plan for you in the Universe. (Dyer, 2006)

Victor is a practical person and clearly speaks what's on his mind. In those seven years, he has gone from being frustrated and pulling tantrums, to having profound emotional intelligence.

N.B. ** It is now important to obtain a Travel Plan (ascia) from your child's doctor to be able to take Adrenaline Autoinjectors (Epi-Pens/ Anapens) on board aeroplanes in hand luggage or on the person.

20. SWIMMING POOLS

'Australia is famous for producing Olympic Swimming Champions. It is of little wonder as we live on an island and are taught to swim from babyhood.'

Summertime in Queensland means heading to the beach or a swimming pool for a swim to cool off. It is a part of our culture and lifestyle.
Pool parties are another common occurrence for adults and children alike.

About a month after Victor's anaphylactic reaction, he was invited to his first birthday pool party. Victor loved the water, so much so, that when he was about three, he'd scaled a friend's swimming pool fence and jumped into the centre of the pool.

In the twinkling of an eye, Victor had climbed the pool fence and jumped into the water. Mid-Winter, the four feet deep pool was icy cold.

On crutches, I had a sprained ankle from playing basketball. My quick-thinking friend, Lisa slipped off her shoes and dove straight in clothes and all.

Lisa saved Victor that day. I am forever thankful for her practical courage. I warmed Victor up slowly in the bath to combat slight hypothermia. Otherwise, he was fine.

After that, though our budget was tight, Victor started swimming lessons and enjoyed them immensely.

When he was invited to the pool party, he instantly wanted to go. I knew he was a good swimmer and capable of saving himself.

However, my first thought was if anyone in the pool had nuts in their mouth from eating food, there was a good chance that the contents of their mouth would be washed out by the pool water. If that was the case, nut allergens could wash into my child's mouth.

Once again, I had to source some information about the likelihood of Victor having an anaphylactic reaction in the pool.

I asked my doctor, rang pool companies and researched on the internet. The consensus was that any potential allergens would be filtered out or killed off by the chlorine. For Victor's sake, I chose to believe it.

Victor was fine at the pool party, enjoying a lengthy swim with his friends.

That year, Victor swam in many people's private pools, large public pools and at the beach.

He had no reaction whatsoever so I assumed it was safe to swim. He has swum happily for many years now.

21. CROSS CONTAMINATION

'When someone makes a sandwich, who can remember how they made it a week later?'

Cross-contamination of food can be a real danger to a person with an allergy. Most cross-contamination I've found, was to do with butter/ margarine and spreads. By using a different knife for each food, and training all of the family and anyone staying at my home, reduction in stress was immense.

Wiping a knife with peanut butter or Nutella with a paper towel and discarding the soiled towel in the rubbish bin, enabled Victor to take his turn washing the dishes, the same as everyone in the family. I also wiped a nut spread coated knife, before placing it in the dishwasher. I purchased more knives so we didn't run out before the dishes were done.

I also decided to allow Victor to eat Australian-made processed foods that didn't actually contain nuts, but were labelled that 'they may contain traces of nuts'.

My sister-in-law, Yvette worked at a biscuit-/ cookie- making factory. She informed me that often, it was months before a nut-based product came through. After each run of biscuits, the machinery was cleaned thoroughly. The label stating that 'the product may contain traces of nuts and/or processed on machinery that uses tree nuts or sesame seeds', was put on packing to cover liability.

I believed that if there were minute amounts of nuts in the air, or on the machines during food processing, this would benefit Victor by re-conditioning his cells not to react as if the nut protein was a major enemy and shut down.

N.B. ** Recently, there has been a move towards food companies labelling their processed foods correctly so people suffering allergies can eat more products not actually made from allergens. This will make things clearer and expand the variety of foods that can be safely eaten.

Another source of cross-contamination was toothpaste. I always made sure that everyone in the family had their own labelled toothbrush and toothpaste. Quite often bits of food can remain in the bristles of toothbrushes, even after rinsing. When applying toothpaste to the brush, there can be draw back into the toothpaste tube so contaminants and allergens can often sit inside the top of the tube. The next person to use the toothpaste could get a dose of whatever is in there. I found by keeping everyone's tooth brushing utensils separate, it also often prevented the spread of colds and flu, throughout the entire family.

Wiping the light switches and door knobs once a week with disinfectant wipes, also helped to reduce cross-contamination.

Being aware of preventing cross-contamination, gives peace of mind and reduces the risk of anaphylactic reaction caused by a break in the chain of asepsis. (Asepsis means a condition where no disease-causing bacteria are present.)

Having been a qualified and practicing School Dental Therapist (now called Oral Health Therapist) for fourteen years, I was well-versed in not transferring bacteria, viruses and allergens from one surface to another or one patient to another.

Maintaining the chain of asepsis works to keep everyone healthy. Being a fanatic though, can cause more stress and weaken the immune system.

22. THE WHOLE SCHOOL THING

'Where else do you get to hang out with your friends every day, but school?'

Attending school is an important part of socialising and learning skills to equip one for life in the big wide world.

There is also bullying to deal with. Bullies often target children that are different and deemed weaker than they are.

In primary/ elementary school, Victor was bullied. He was behind with his speech development. He was underweight. He also had a nut allergy. Because of the delayed speech, it was difficult to make friends. He was pushed into the garden and his arm was broken.

In some ways, not making friends easily went in his favour, as he didn't swap food with other kids at recess/ First Break, or lunch time/ Second Break.

Of course, all that changed after a few years, when he could speak well. Often he would come home with chocolate bar wrappers in his lunch box. They had print on them in a foreign language. That was daunting. Sometimes, it would happen every day for a week. Eventually, I figured that he wasn't having a reaction to it and relaxed about it. What was more important was that he'd made a friend.

I would remind him not to swap food at school. However, that seemed to be forgotten once at school. I made his teachers aware of it. They reminded him, but like a lot of things that are out of your control, I had to weigh up the positives and go with the flow.

Another source of potential cross-contamination was putting his mouth on shared bubblers at the drinking troughs. Again, it was something beyond my control. I would always pack a bottle of purified water with his lunch box. I would then ask him to drink only from it and to stay away from the bubblers, but that too often fell on deaf ears.

When a teacher says to the class after a Physical Education lesson to go get a drink, nine times out of ten, like a pack of wild horses, they will all gallop towards the bubblers.

As the Epi-Pen Junior/ Epi-Pen was kept inside Victor's classroom, the highest risk times were in the playground at lunch time, when other teachers were on duty. If he was playing on the oval, it was also a fair distance away from where the Epi-Pen Junior/ Epi-Pen was located. I decided that if he was going to have an anaphylactic reaction, it would more likely happen, when he was eating rather than playing, so I relaxed about this.

By packing a healthy lunch with some treats, Victor was more likely to eat it and thus, prevent a reaction. Victor knew to bring home the wrappers of what he had eaten, so I could see, what he preferred to eat most often.

When opportunities came up for him to play interschool sport, I encouraged it. He needed a chance to dream, create and achieve like any other child. I always reminded his teachers the morning of the interschool sports day to take his Epi-Pen Junior/ Epi-Pen on the bus.

By Grade Three, Victor was ready to go on a three day excursion to Camp Curramundi. It was a fabulous place boasting all kinds of exciting outdoor activities, from tree-top rope walks, abseiling down walls and raft building.

Nervous to let him stay for three days with mass- produced camp food, I was able to call and talk with the chef. She very kindly offered to make him foods that he liked and could eat, cooking them in separate pans. I decided to go with him on his first camp, as a parent volunteer. There were several children with various allergies and I ended up looking after them all. Everyone with an allergy had brought their own food with them, so it made it very easy to feed these kids. Victor and I had a ball!

Every year after that, he went on camp without me. Sometimes, a teacher would ring me and ask why I'd packed so much food. I was always worried that he'd starve, which in hindsight was just 'fear of the unknown' talking doom and gloom in my head.

In the end, I didn't pack any food, because most of it was being wasted. He survived, albeit, he always came home tired with a cold and needed a couple of day's bed rest like most of the other children.

By the time, he was in Sixth Grade; he was eligible to go on a Snowy Mountains Trip, away for seven days. Scary stuff, but I remained upbeat and positive. It was good for his independence, to rely on himself to take care and see more of the world, I told myself. And it was. He saw snow for the first time; learned to ski; saw our nation's Capital; and enjoyed himself immensely with his friends.

High school was a different kettle of fish. Victor was the little fish again in a big pond. He had to move around. Go from class to class. Teacher to teacher.

He needed a new strategy for survival. His Epi-Pen was kept in his backpack. He needed to be confident in how to use it himself. I'd read that students with nut allergies carried mobile/ cell phones with a speed dial to the school's office, so they could say where they were. Then, the office personnel could ring the paramedics and direct them to where he was in the school, as quickly as possible.

I refrained from buying a mobile/ cell phone. They were expensive to maintain and also frowned upon at the High School, because they often interfered with the learning in class and were a temptation for potential cyber-bullying.

Instead, I met with the Deputy Principal to advise them of Victor's anaphylactic nut allergy. The Deputy Principal informed me that, as mandatory Duty of Care, all staff were now trained in the administration of the Epi-Pen and knew to call the paramedics immediately. Victor's friends also knew to get a teacher in a hurry, if he had an anaphylactic reaction outside of the classroom.

Again, starting a new school where many students didn't know him was a concern. Teenagers were often bullied and did thoughtless things, when hormones were fuelling their impulses. Would one of them take a dislike to him and shove peanut butter down his throat? Would they do it for a joke or a dare or just to see what would happen?

Thankfully, I found that none of these things ever happened. I sent Victor to the High School, where most of his friends were going. This offered protection within a pack.

Luckily, Victor wasn't girl crazy. He preferred to hang out with his mates. Both Adam and I were late bloomers; Freddie also seemed to be, so we hoped Victor would be too.

But when girl fever and sex naturally occurred, I had to prepare him well.

23. DATING

'Falling in love is the most wonderful time of your life.'

From an early age, I always talked to my children about relationships. Even before, the inevitable 'sex talks', I discussed the value in maintaining good, long-term friendships.

It was important to be kind, considerate and compassionate. To give and to receive unconditionally. Character traits such as: trustworthiness; honesty; loyalty; respect and taking responsibility for one's own actions were also keys in developing as a person, as well as being a good citizen in society.

Working for several years at a High School, many girls would confide in me, that they'd had sex from an early age, often before they'd started High School. Many boys did too, but they seemed to start two or three years later than the girls.

My boys seemed more studiously inclined and were interested in music and sport. But then again, I'd always stressed that it was better to wait until they were adults, make friends and get to know people, before embarking on the intimacy of intercourse.

Nowadays, the hormones of puberty can kick in from as young as nine years of age. Hence, I believed it was imperative to talk to Victor often about different scenarios, where his life could be put in danger.

A headline in the newspaper grabbed my attention one day where a teenage boy with an anaphylactic nut allergy had died, after his girlfriend had kissed him. It happened at school, four hours after she'd had a nut cereal for breakfast. It was a very sad turn of events for the boy and his girlfriend and their families.

I let Victor know about it and we discussed ways of preventing this from happening.

At first, Victor said that he wouldn't have any relationships. He would live alone all his adult life.

I told him that that was an option, but not ideal, as loving someone was a wonderful experience. Companionship and making love were two very enjoyable pastimes in life. It was also often necessary to have children.

Though he had no thoughts of having children, as the puberty hormones kicked in, he started to understand what I was taking about.

What we came up with was:
* Trust was a big issue in forming relationships.
* Love and caring would have to be exhibited before kissing anyone.
* Much communication would be needed before kissing anyone.
* It was better to form a relationship with someone who had natural

beauty inside and out, than with someone who liked to wear make-up. (Foundation and lipstick often contain nut oils.)

- The girlfriend/ boyfriend would need to be aware of the nut allergy and consequences and would need to kindly refrain from eating nuts/ nut products, during their relationship.
- My child had to be forthright and practical. If the potential partner wasn't prepared to consider his needs, he needed to remain friends or part company. It was as simple as that. Intimacy wasn't possible.

Easy to say, but sometimes, difficult to do especially when sexual attraction is intense.

Again, this aspect of Victor's life was something out of my control. Once he became an adult, he would be captain of his own ship. He had to make his own choices in life and reap the rewards or suffer the consequences. My job as a mother was to teach him as much as possible about life, so he could function well in the big wide world.

I would often say, in the ideal world, if he met a partner who also had a nut allergy, then they would understand each other's dietary and health needs perfectly.

Adam and I have always eaten nuts/ nut products every day. We have always given our children lots of kisses on their skin and hugs. Victor has always been fine.

As the skin was an organ of the body, perhaps by kissing it, I believed it would help him build up a tolerance to the nut protein.

As Victor hasn't fallen in love yet or kissed a girl or boy (you never know these days), it hasn't been an issue.

I'm sure one day, it will come. All I've asked him to do was to remember the Scout's motto: Always Be Prepared!

24. NIGHT CLUBBING

'Move over Drugs, Sex and Rock'n'Roll. Dancing, drinking, brawling and hooking up are often what teenage dreams are made of.'

Part of the rite of passage in many cultures is to have their first taste of alcohol at eighteen.

Unfortunately, in reality, this often occurs much earlier. Though Adam and I seldom drink alcohol, we still remember those carefree years of our late teens and early twenties, when going to parties and night clubs was a ritual, almost every weekend. They were fun, exciting and often spontaneous times.

Times have changed now where drugs are more varied and prevalent; alcohol is served in plastic cups to prevent many injuries, when violence erupts; and Sexually Transmitted Infections (STI's) can seriously affect your health, or be deadly in the form of AIDS.

Adam and I have always encouraged our children to find their natural talents and to follow their dreams. If going to parties and night clubs was part of their journey, then so be it.

Besides the usual warnings about the consequences of risky behaviour in the form of drink or drug driving; fighting; and unsafe sex; I recommended that Victor needed to avoid "Shouts". "Shouts" are when everyone in the group takes turns at buying a round of drinks for everyone else. It's very expensive as well as a way of accelerating drunkenness.

My main concern to him was that eating nuts often went with drinking beer. Sometimes, they're in bowls on the bar. Someone could easily contaminate a drink or glass unwittingly, with nut protein residue. As people drink more, the rational side of their brain becomes impaired, so I made Victor aware of what would happen if he drank.

Besides, the risk of someone spiking his drink with a drug, it was better if he bought and kept hold of his drinks at all times, to lessen or eliminate the chance of nut protein contamination.

I even tell my children to finish their drink before they go to the toilet and buy a new one later. Leaving their drink with a trusted friend is no guarantee that the drink won't be spiked or contaminated. The friend could become distracted, or be too inebriated to be mindful of the importance to take care of it.

In the end, my children had to learn to look after of themselves.

THE PHYSICAL ELEMENTS

'For every action in the Universe, there is an opposing reaction. What if one stopped resisting the reaction and went with the flow? Would that in itself be healing enough?'

THE MEDICAL CONDITION

There are many theories put forward how a nut allergy occurs. Everything from mothers eating nuts while pregnant; to depletion of nutrients in the soil; to parents not allowing their children to play in the dirt; to genetically-engineered foods; to highly-processed foods and a vast array of additives and preservatives that have altered our DNA; to people building up a tolerance to food from eating too much of it; to the over-use of antibiotics; or perhaps, some or all of the above.

So far, there still doesn't seem to be a proven, specific cause. All we know is that food and drug allergies and intolerances seem to be more prevalent in the modern age. One recent study has shown that the peanut allergy has only manifested in society since the introduction of genetically-modified peanuts. With over 20% of our youth living with a nut allergy on a global scale, that in effect, means millions are being affected.

Mentally, I went through all the theories of the physical manifestation of anaphylactic reaction. In effect, an alien substance enters the body and causes antibodies to go into immediate attack mode. They shut down cellular matter. For something to override our body's natural tendency for self-preservation, I came to the conclusion that there must be more to it. Nut Allergy appears to be an Auto Immune Disease, which I interpreted as the immune system had somehow decided to automatically dysfunction on purpose.

The automatic or parasympathetic side of the brain unconsciously keeps us breathing; our heart beating; and our endocrine or glandular system, providing lymphatic cells to fight any bacteria or viruses that enter our body.

Why would the mind choose to ruin its survival coding?

A.I.D.S. – AUTO IMMUNE DISEASE SIGNIFICANCE

From my observations and life experience, it seems likely that a thought pattern behind attracting A.I.D.S. to oneself could stem from being in denial of who you are. It can also be from sexual guilt or not believing that you are good enough. (Hay, 1984)

I began to think how could young people be thinking like this? Was my child unconsciously sabotaging himself? What did 'being in denial of who you are' mean anyhow? Could someone so young not want to live on the Earth? In their own skin? Was life too sped up for them? Was the breakdown in family units and community ties making them not want to live long enough to explore the world and find out who they were as a growing and developing human being?

Was there a sensory overload with too much technology? Watching DVD's over and over, playing computer games, did they have some sort of adverse effect? Did it kill their passion? Did they make them think that life was the same all the time? Repetitive - like being on a merry-go-round? Did they secretly want to get off that merry-go-round? Or did it make them think that life was supposed to be exciting 24/7? That boredom and relaxing by doing nothing at all, wasn't a part of modern life.

Did we, as parents, push them to achieve in various sporting, artistic or academic fields too hard and too soon?

Could they feel guilty about their sexuality? What if they were told it was bad or dirty to fondle their genitals when they were little, when it gave them infinite pleasure?

What if they were always being corrected, when they tried to do something for the first time, or stopped from exploring their world freely? Would that affect how they felt about themselves? Would they feel not good enough, that they had to be perfect?

Maybe, being perfect was too hard, so they decided to shut down their little bodies and try to escape the pressure.

From my observations and life experience, allergies seemed to be caused by a thought pattern of denying your own power. People could also be allergic or reacting adversely to someone close to them. (Hay, 1994)

Could children feel unsure of themselves being thrown into a school system, where right from five years of age, or sometimes earlier, they are made to attend an alien place, where they had to keep busy inputting knowledge for five hours, five days a week? Prep students now get homework and assignments to do.

Some countries start their children at school at age seven. I wondered if they have a lessened incidence of allergies in those children. Studies needed to be done.

From my observations and life experience, breathing problems seemed to be caused by a thought pattern of fear or of not wanting to experience all aspects of life. It could also be from feeling important enough to be here or even exist. (Hay, 1984)

I began to wonder, did position in the family have an effect on their self-esteem? Did they have a stubborn streak? Did they feel unworthy of being loved, for who they were?

Victor has had a bout every Winter of Impetigo (School Sores), since starting school. Was his body manifesting that school didn't agree with him? He has always hated school with a passion. He had often said that it was boring, repetitive and most of the knowledge was useless. He believed that if he wanted to know something, he'd look it up on the internet. Was he rebelling against the school system? Spending so much of his life there, then having to do homework, was it eating at the very fibre of his being? He'd always complained that there was too much homework and not enough fun time.

A human being is a very complex, unique organism. Not only is the functioning of the physical body a miraculous piece of creation, it also has an ever-expanding mind and soul.

THE EMOTIONAL ELEMENTS

'When emotions are pushed down, they stay in the body until they are allowed to be expressed freely.'

An allergy is not a normal response or reaction. It may occur when someone or something is bothering you over a period of time. It can spring from someone overreacting emotionally and not being honest with how upsetting it is. By not setting boundaries within you and with others, one can feel annoyed and powerless. It appears to come from being emotional and not true to your feelings. (Noontil, 1994)

Could Victor's feelings have affected the way his body was functioning? I needed to explore this idea further.

Through extensive reading, I discovered that emotions are carried around in our bodies by small proteins called, Peptides. They are programmed by the way we think. (Chopra, 1998)

When dis-ease (negative thought patterns) lodges in the body, it can cause many of the illnesses we see manifested in humans today.

Auto Immune Disease Syndromes may affect the parts of your body that you have weakened by your negative internal thoughts. When your inner-peace is shattered, the auto immune system gives up its defence mechanisms. Therefore, it is important to be fully involved in all aspects of life. Being fulfilled and successful can obliterate those self-destructive thoughts. (Noontil, 1994)

As a child is growing and developing in the modern world, it takes time to gain knowledge, life experience and to feel confident in one's own skin. Often children believe what adults and other children say they are. Negative comments can hurt and stay in a child's memory forever. By letting others dictate the way they think about themselves, a child can become powerless and experience low self-esteem.

Praise and unconditional encouragement are ways parents can help their children feel good about themselves. The children can then feel nurtured and able to explore the world to find their true selves and natural talents. Children can love themselves regardless of what other people say or think they are thinking.

If they are only taught about the physical things in life like having money and owning things, then they are not growing in spirit. They will not have inner-peace nor will they follow their soul plan. Feelings of not wanting to be here can arise from this and the immune system can be compromised.

(Noontil, 1994)

At school, Victor was often bullied in those early years. He couldn't speak very well, so he was hard to understand. Anger and frustration would often grip him. In Preschool (now Prep), he was sent to a Special School to be with a small group of boys, who needed more immersion in language. Though the staff was very lovely and compassionate, he often came home frustrated because he missed his Preschool friends.

On the opposite side of the coin, Victor was gifted in the area of Mathematics. For Maths, his Preschool Teacher planned to send him and his friend into a Grade 1, 2, 3 Composite Class (60 students) once a week. On the first day, they didn't last more than ten minutes, before they ran out of the classroom and jumped the fence back into Preschool. I believe they were overwhelmed by the whole experience. It was a case of too much, too soon!

When Victor was in Grade Two, one of his teachers was teaching him advanced, lateral-thinking Maths. This happened before he had his anaphylactic reaction. Maybe, it was too intense for him once again.

The more I became aware of what Victor may be experiencing in his everyday life, the sooner I realised that his inner-feelings, were often overloaded. That his sensors being constantly overwhelmed. Was adrenaline being constantly pumped through his body? Did that make his system want to shut down?

Was it really necessary to keep children super-busy all the time?

THE ROLE OF FEAR AND ANXIETY

Most people have a fear of death. It usually starts during puberty, when teenagers are finding who they are and where they fit into the world. They often perceive that they are invincible. When a beloved pet or someone close or related dies and doesn't return, a fear of death appears to remain latent in the subconscious.

However, when a child has an anaphylactic reaction prior to puberty, when they have almost died, the fear of death can kick in earlier. Subsequently, if other anaphylactic reactions start occurring, cell memory brings the fear of death into the conscious mind. The body reacts by either fight or flight. Both reactions send nor-adrenaline from the brain into the blood stream. This release acts like a catalyst, which rapidly increases the heart beat to send blood to muscles. In consequence, the anaphylactic reaction also happens faster.

Fear of the unknown is basically worry. Worrying about something that may never come, wastes energy. Worry seems to also begat more worry, until the brain cannot switch off from it. If habitual, it could be classed as a form of self-abuse.

If an anaphylactic reaction does start to exhibit signs and symptoms in the body such as: Hives or Welts; Wheezing or difficulty Breathing; or Facial Swelling, remaining calm seems to slow the reaction down considerably.

Anxiety is caused by fear. One of the main symptoms of anxiety is shortness of breath.

When someone wheezes, they are complaining to themselves that they aren't allowed to do things their way. (Noontil, 1994)

Children have their individual personality traits right from birth. It is important to take a step back and understand that children may learn differently and like to do things differently. Some children learn from seeing how things are done; listening to or reading instructions; or working it out and doing it by themselves.

Children learn from their environment, their experiences and the way parents display their parenting skills. Love is a given, but also how parents were brought up as children, plays a part in their own parenting styles.

I found quite often I would repeat a saying, or mimic an action; my parents said or did to me in my childhood. Some were positive influences on me and others were negative.

Deciding to parent my children differently to the way I was brought up, took courage and dedication. It was easy to slip back into old, familiar patterns, especially when my husband and his parents, were parented differently again.

Consistency, I realised, was the best way to bring up children, so they didn't get mixed messages and become confused, or play one parent against the other.

For my own knowledge, I read many parenting books; examined my children's astrological birth chart to understand their different natures; and attended parenting courses, when offered at my children's schools.

Nothing can really prepare you for parenting. In this ever-changing world, I believe it is the hardest job on Earth. As children grow and learn and form their own opinions, parents are required to keep abreast with the changes, while earning a living. As more siblings are born, which makes all the children continuously at different stages in the family, re-evaluation of parenting strategies is not only crucial, but a necessity. If family values and ethics are healthy and strong, dysfunction usually doesn't occur, but that doesn't stop adversity coming from outside influences.

Being fearless can be dangerous, but being risk-less, keeps people from moving forward successfully and in the case of Nut Allergy, it puts a barrier in the way of healing completely.

By removing the barrier, the journey of returning to normal health can begin.

SELF-ESTEEM AND SELF-CONFIDENCE

When one doesn't love themselves enough to enjoy life, they cannot enjoy it fully or properly.

If the child learns to love themselves and feel good about themselves, then regular breathing will become the norm. (Noontil, 1994)

To improve Victor's self-esteem, self-confidence and self-worth, I proactively did several things. They included:

1. I loved him unconditionally for whom or what he was.
2. I refrained from comparing him to his brother or any other child in any way.
3. I read to him many children's books and listened to him read to me with praise.
4. I slowed everything down from how fast I normally talked, to giving him the time he needed to learn a new skill, listening.
5. I spent equal quality time with each child.
6. I played lots of board games and cards with him.
7. I managed his football (soccer) team for many years.
8. I encouraged him to enter Football Carnivals to experience the joy of winning and the disappointment of losing.
9. I taught him how to do housework and cook for himself.
10. Adam taught him to mow the lawn.
11. We often played Backyard Cricket together as a family.
12. I encouraged him to try new things, to find his natural talent and take responsibility for his own actions.

Adam built Victor a trophy cabinet, for all his participation trophies and medals. On his bedroom walls, I put up team photos and awards he received at school.

His teachers often gave out classroom awards for improvements in handwriting; social skills and co-operation. They were also laminated and went on his walls.

By making commitments to playing in a sporting team, chess team and instrumental school band for a year at a time, perseverance, resilience and the importance of mastering a skill were learned and enjoyed by him. If he liked the vocation, he would stick at it for many years, to become competent and in consequence, successful.

Knowing he was part of a bigger picture or team increased his realisation that he was important, like an integral part of an eco-system.

As a football/ cricket manager, I made sure that every child in each team received the same amount of encouragement awards. I always wrote on them something positive that they'd achieved in the game, or a skill on which they had improved. By doing that, all of the team appreciated one another and their self-worth and esteem was highlighted. All of the team became self-confident and happily continue to play team sports today. Many have gone on to represent their Region, State and Country.

It's not about winning every game. There can only be one winner in competitive sports. It's Win-Win, if the players have given it their all and enjoyed themselves. They can then take that attitude and strength of character into all areas of their lives.

To change negative thought patterns, I removed the words, 'should' and 'ought to' from my vocabulary. I replaced them with 'prefer' or 'may choose to'. I also let go of the outcome.

I only give out advice when it asked for. Whether or not, it is taken up now, later, or never, is the choice of the receiver.

I chose to remove the word, 'Don't' from my vocabulary, as well. It seems that children do not hear the word 'Don't' e.g. 'Don't run away.' They run away and we, as parents, become angry.

By saying it in a positive way e.g. 'Stay here.' They stay put and we praise them.

It's as simple as that. Most children want to please their parents. It's a Win-Win situation and everyone's happy.

Help them to discover their natural talents, by noting what they are doing for play. Encourage and nurture those interests.

Victor liked: building with Lego; writing lists of numbers; reading story books; watching 'Teletubbies', 'Mathematician' and 'The Thunderbirds'; painting; colouring in; climbing trees, (Fences and the garage roof! He was very sure-footed.); playing cards and 'Monopoly'; swimming; dancing; singing; riding his bicycle; running; playing with balls; playing toy musical instruments; telling jokes and making up funny songs (parodies).

When older, he liked: writing out sports statistics; budgeting to buy something with the pocket money he'd earned from doing weekly household chores; playing Xbox and computer games; playing with his dog; playing club football (soccer), cricket and various interschool sports; Paintball, Laser force and Ten Pin Bowling; riding his bicycle exploring the neighbourhood; watching humorous skits and parodies on 'You Tube'; and chatting with his mates on 'Skype', while playing interactive Live Team games.

Children still need boundaries and are governed to engage in some form of education, either at Private, Public, Distance or Home Schools. If their hobbies and interests fulfil them, they are happier to exist in the world and are more resilient during times of adversity. Having something else to think about also keeps fear away.

THE MENTAL ELEMENTS

'Denying of the Will may lead to blocking of the life force and in consequence, cause death.'

When a baby is born, their mind is a clean slate. They have some experiences already in the womb, as they are intrinsically connected to their mother's mind and her experiences in cell memory and environment, during pregnancy.

I was happy at home raising and playing with my son, Freddie, who liked to do a great variety of activities each day. At thirty-eight, I also was happy to have fallen pregnant a second time, after trying for a year.
My husband, Adam had wanted one child. I had wanted three. As we were older parents, we compromised with two.

On each day of my second pregnancy, to my surprise, I had spontaneous orgasms. I only mention this, as I didn't experience these phenomena with my first pregnancy. Perhaps, this may prove to be a common link with other women, who have children who have developed allergies. Please let me know.

A.I.D.S. also affects the third chakra (sexual/ creative chakra), so perhaps, Victor was constantly in a blissful, orgasmic state in the womb and being born into the real world wasn't the same, or a big comedown (excuse the pun!)

Could this have caused a malfunction in his body, mind and soul? Perhaps, a study could be done.

In the first five years, learning and growing as a human being, a baby absorbs an incredible amount of information on all levels - physical, emotional, mental and spiritual.

On the mental level, understanding body language, speech patterns and whether their basic needs for wellness are being meet, are all being molded in their developing brains from the get-go.

It was discovered that babies (0-3 months) have five distinct cries; their way of communicating their needs. They are:

1. "Neh" - The need for nourishment;

2. "Heh" - The need for love (touch, emotional comfort, interaction, being bored, or overwhelmed) and nappy/ diaper change (physical comfort);

3. "Owh" - The need for sleep;

4. "Eairh" - The need for pain relief e.g. Colic/ lower gas; and

5. "Eh" – The need to burp after having a breast or bottle milk feed. (Dunstan, www.parenthood.com, 14th January, 2014).

It has been proven that all babies regardless of nationality or culture respond this way. Therefore, it is safe to say that these responses are automatic. Does the baby think about their needs before they cry? In the gap between registering the thought in the brain and the subsequent response, they probably do - if only for a nano-second.

As the baby moves into the toddler stage, they often have recurrent dreams and imaginary friends. They are learning about their environment through their five senses - touch, smell, taste, hearing and sight. Their personality starts to form. They often fall into one of four categories of personality traits - sanguine, phlegmatic, melancholic or choleric.

SANGUINE PERSONALITY

The Sanguine personality is the Extrovert, the Talker, and the Optimist. They win popularity contests and shine like the sun.

As babies, Sanguine Personalities are:
Bright and wide-eyed, curious, gurgle and coo a lot;
Show off;
Are responsive;
Often scream for attention; and
Know they are cute.

As children, Sanguine Personalities are:
Daring and eager;
Innocent;
Inventive, imaginative and can tell fibs;
Cheerful and easily distracted;
Enthusiastic, energised and fun-loving;
Chatter constantly and be forgetful; and
Can bounce back from adversity quickly.

As teenagers, Sanguine Personalities are:
Are cheerleaders, get daring and join clubs;
Charm others;
Are creative, deceptive and make elaborate excuses;
Be the life of the party;
Need peer approval and like to gossip;
Crave attention; and
Can shirk study and responsibility.

Emotionally, they need attention, approval, affection, acceptance, people around them, and activity. They often avoid dull tasks, routines, criticism, details, and lofty goals.

PHLEGMATIC PERSONALITY

The Phlegmatic personality is the Introvert, the Follower, and the Pessimist. They are calm and enjoy peace and quiet. They are stable and down-to-earth like a country meadow.

As babies, Phlegmatic Personalities are:
Easy-going, undemanding and happy;
Adjustable;
Slow;
Shy; and
Indifferent.

As children, Phlegmatic Personalities are:
Observant of others;
Easily amused;
Cause little trouble but can avoid work;
Dependable;
Lovable but can be lazy;
Agreeable, fearful, quietly stubborn and can retreat to technologies; and
Can be selfish and tease others.

As teenagers, Phlegmatic Personalities are:
Leaders when pushed;
Have pleasing personalities;
Are witty and a good listener;
Can be too compromising;
Mediate problems;
Be unenthusiastic and indecisive;
Can hide emotions, quietly stubborn and have a casual attitude; and
Can be unmotivated, sarcastic, uninvolved and can procrastinate.

Emotionally, they need peace and relaxation, attention, praise, self-worth and loving motivation. They also need to avoid conflict, confrontations, initiative, decisions, extra work, responsibility, tensions and quarrels.

MELANCHOLIC PERSONALITY

The Melancholic personality is the Introvert, the Thinker, and the Pessimist. They are perfectionists and their psyche is complex and unfathomable like the deepest part of the ocean.

As babies, Melancholic Personalities are:
Serious, quiet and clingy;
Like a schedule;
Look sad;
Cry easily.

As children, Melancholic Personalities are:
Deep thinkers, are intense, dutiful and responsible;
Are talented, sensitive and musical;
Are perfectionists and avoid criticism;
Daydream, always see a problem and hear a negative;
Are moody, whine a lot, can be self-conscious, won't communicate; and
Be a true friend.

As teenagers, Melancholic Personalities are:
Studious, creative and like to research;
Are organised, purposeful but may have a negative attitude;
Have a poor self-image and can be revengeful;
Have high standards, are conscientious and on time, neat and orderly;
Can be depressed, withdrawn and have an inferiority complex;
Can be inflexible, be suspicious of people and be critical;
Are sensitive to others needs, have a sweet spirit and are thrifty;
May live their life through their friends and need approval.

Emotionally, they need sensitivity to deep desires; satisfaction from quality achievement; space to call their own; security and stability; separation from noisy, messy siblings; and support from their parents: 'I believe in you.' They also avoid noise, confusion, trivial pursuits and being cheered up.

CHOLERIC PERSONALITY

The Choleric personality is the Extrovert, the Leader, and the Optimist. They are powerful and fierce like the fire storms of the Sun. The size of the fire storm depends on how it is managed.

As babies, Choleric Personalities are:
Adventuresome, Outgoing and Precocious;
A Born Leader;
Strong-willed, loud and demanding; and
Throw things and avoid sleep to gain more attention.

As children, Choleric Personalities are:
Daring and eager;
Can see a goal and move quickly;
Are constantly on-the-go;
Are self-sufficient and trustworthy;
Can be manipulative and throw tantrums;
Are competitive and assertive;
Insistent, testing and argumentative; and
Stubborn and determined.

As teenagers, Choleric Personalities are:
Aggressive and competent;
Are self-confident and stimulate others;
Excel in emergencies, have great potential and are responsible;
Can be too bossy, control parents, be know-it-alls, and be superior;
Organise well, assume leadership roles and can problem solve;
Can be unpopular and become a loner; and
Can be insulting, judgmental and unrepentant.

Emotionally, they need appreciation for all their achievements, opportunity for leadership, participation in family decisions, something to control, their own room, garage, backyard, and/ or dog. They like to avoid rest, boredom and playing games that they cannot win!

ASTROLOGICAL SIGNS

Often the personality traits line up with their astrological and elemental group. This is often a good place to start understanding your child. The elemental groups are: Air, Water, Earth and Fire.

AIR SIGNS

The Air signs are: Libra (September 23rd - October 22nd); Gemini (May 23rd - June 22nd); and Aquarius (January 23rd - February 22nd). With over thirty years' experience, I can confidently say that they are often, more than not, Sanguine in personality.

WATER SIGNS

The Water signs are: Cancer (June 23rd - July 22nd); Scorpio (October 23rd - November 22nd); and Pisces (February 23rd - March 22nd). I can confidently say that they are, often more than not, Melancholic in personality.

EARTH SIGNS

The Earth signs are: Capricorn (December 23rd - January 22nd); Taurus (April 23rd - May 22nd); and Virgo (August 23rd - September 22nd). I can confidently say that they are, often more than not, Phlegmatic in personality.

FIRE SIGNS

The Fire signs Are: Aries (March 23rd - April 22nd); Leo (July 23rd - August 22nd); and Sagittarius (November 23rd - December 22nd). I can confidently say that they are, often more than not, Choleric in personality.

Within the elements of Air, Water, Earth and Fire, there are also three sub-groups: Cardinal (like to lead); Fixed (like to stand their ground); and Mutable (like to go with the flow). These also affect personality and give the different nuances in behaviour.

Children's behaviours are believed to be a mix of four influences: temperament; parenting style; reaction to stress and uncertainty; and the pursuit of attention and power. Position in the family also affects these influences to varying degrees. (Green, 2000)

Having studied astrology for over thirty years, individual birth charts are more accurate and specific for understanding the uniqueness of your child on their journey through life. Cherishing each child for their individuality without comparison, is a way of parenting which I believe, increases their self-esteem and self-worth. It's important to remember that siblings are always at different developmental stages right through until they become adults.

Victor is a phlegmatic type personality and a staunch advocate for fairness. From an early age, he liked to do things on his own. When he was passionate about something, he would focus on it for a long time. Having an enthusiastic penchant for watching football on television, he would frequently write out orderly lists of football statistics from the Sunday newspaper. He received lots of praise for his efforts. He stopped doing this around the age of ten, when he began appearing in the Sunday newspaper in the cricket statistics. Perhaps, he'd realised his goal.

By encouraging his positive personality strengths and gently redirecting his negative weaknesses, Victor has become mentally resilient and has developed into a confident young man.

Both emotional and mental intelligence is important, when embarking as an adult into today's big, wide world.

MY CHILD IS NOT A NUT ALLERGY

'Labels are for peanut butter jars, not people!'

From the day Victor was first diagnosed by the doctor, he was often seen as a walking, breathing, eating Nut Allergy. He ceased being a normal seven year old boy and became the allergy in many people's eyes.

Many people were afraid of him, as if they could catch something deadly from him, or that if they went near him, he could drop dead right before their eyes.

It took quite a while to convince and educate people that indeed, Victor still was that loveable, perky bright spark of a person they all knew and liked. With prevention, he wasn't going to stop breathing in the classroom, on the street or in other people's homes.

I was exhausted emotionally due to shock and fear, but I soon realised that many people lived with all kinds of afflictions - physical, emotional and mental. There were far worse afflictions out there.
For Victor's Grade 3, 4 & 5 teachers, I chose a teacher who had previously been a competitive swimmer and nurse, before studying teaching.

I recall Victor's first words to her were, 'I am a nut. I have rubber butt. Every time I turn around, it goes putt-putt.' Even then, Victor had a Jim Carrey-like sense of humour.

His teacher laughed and said, 'I like kids with a bit of spunk.'
I could have hugged her. She was the first person to whom I'd told that Victor had a nut allergy, outside my immediate family and friends, who didn't take two steps back.

After that encounter, I knew Victor had a decent chance of having a normal life and making it in the world.

LIVING WELL

'By removing lust, hatred and ignorance from our psyche, one can be enlightened with the truth of living well.'

For anyone living in the new millennium, the importance of keeping one's mental health is vital to living a full and enjoyable life.

With the threat of terrorism; the social and financial impact of the internet; medical break-throughs that enable people to live longer; the sustainability of the planet with a huge and growing population; the increase in natural disasters; the destabilisation of many countries; and the breakdown of traditional family and religious values, it is easy for people to become stressed, get the blues or sink into depression.

Having a nut allergy, can only add to all this. For this reason, I have not watched the News for some thirty years. I listen to snippets of the bare facts on the radio, driving to work and skim the headlines of the Sunday newspaper. My family and friends often also give me basic reports on news that affects everyone on the planet.

In consequence, I limit the amount of news that my children see, as often more than not, the opinion or viewpoint of the newsreader/ journalist/ reporter/ media group colours the information.

Victor likes to read the Sports Section of the newspaper. Occasionally, he'll watch a morning program on the television, which tells of the daily news, but is interspersed with light entertainment.

Freddie hears about news through his friends, or on the internet, and Adam reads the newspaper from cover to cover each day.

We tend to listen to music, watch comedy television shows and movies.

We laugh a lot. Learning to clear the mind (meditation), forming one's own philosophies on life and remaining calm to ride the ups and downs of life, enables us all to stay sane.

Love, compassion and belief in oneself are ways to enable one to stay mentally healthy, living with a Nut Allergy and learning to heal.

As it is often said, 'Laughter is the best medicine.'

BEING AND ENJOYING THE MOMENT

'There is only now. Be grateful for the moment and choose to enjoy it.'

Life is made up of moment-by-moment building blocks. By being grateful for every moment in life, it is relative and irrelevant how long we live. By being the best person we can be, by giving to and receiving from the world, our lives hold meaning and balance. By simplifying and becoming aware of each moment, clarification or enlightenment ensues.

Each moment becomes enjoyable. When you are in a state of joy, adversity is less likely to be drawn to or attached to you. Even if adversity comes, by paying attention to it moment-by-moment, it becomes lessened. Often people become overwhelmed by adversity; they attach to it and ride with it down into a negative abyss.

Victor would often come home from school in a grumpy mood.

'How was your day?' I would say.

He would then blurt out, 'It was bad, bad, bad! It just kept getting worse, worse and worse. It's the worst day of my life. . .' And on it went until he was right down there in a negative abyss.

Patiently, I would ask him to break the day down. We would talk through each thing that happened in turn, until he could see everything clearly. He would realise his day wasn't the worst on record; a lot of it boiled down to point of view - his and other people's around him.

Learning to stay in the moment gradually helped him to lessen the chaos. As he became more in control of his thoughts and emotions, enjoying the day was readily possible and happened more frequently.

He became aware of his existence; how his thoughts, actions and reactions directly affected how his day panned out.

Once he became responsible for his actions, reactions were minimised and adversity disappeared.

There were no bad days, because each moment of the day was in the process of change. His perception of the world had changed.

Reality is in the eye of the beholder. According to the laws of Quantum Physics, reality could be real, or it could be an illusion.

Everyone chooses how they perceive something. It's really as simple as that. Magicians have known this for years.

Everything can change in the twinkling of an eye. How you've perceived it, makes all the difference to your action, reaction, or neutral response.

THE SPIRITUAL ELEMENTS

'If you stay the same in mind, body and spirit, that's what you will get is more of the same mind, body and spirit.'

If judgement is released completely, reality can rapidly change. Where there is pure love, no judgement can exist. (Dalai Lama, 2013)

I believe Victor attracted the Nut Allergy to him because he didn't want to live the way he was living anymore. He'd lived the first seven year physical cycle on the planet and realised it wasn't for him. He had also become somewhat disconnected from his father, when Adam started to alternate working two weeks on day shift and two weeks on night shift to earn more money. Adam was the main wage earner; with the increase in the cost of living, he had little choice but to work these hours. The reality was that Adam was available one week out of four, as his body clock was severely affected and he was tired more often than not.

The gaps in Victor's thoughts may have been filled with rage, where he denied himself receiving and giving expressions of love.

As his mother, I filled most of his emotional needs, but during those formative years, he missed a lot of masculine energy. For that reason, he would often crawl into our bed in the middle of the night and sleep between us. As he grew, both Adam and I received our fair share of kicks and head butts.

The fact that Victor had had swelling and inflammation of his face and Epiglottis, when he'd had his anaphylactic reaction seemed to exhibit that there were blockages in his aura relating to self-image and self-expression. Perhaps, he was alternating between feeling loved and unloved. I remember this feeling when growing up. The confusion may have caused the blockages, or deeply embedded it in his soul.

At three and half, Victor was baptised. He screamed over and over. 'No! No! No!' Everyone laughed and the Bishop's nerves were frazzled, but even then he was rebelling against connection with Divine Love.

Did being baptised against his will affect his ability to be heard? Did his spirit give up that day? Or was it just purely fear of the unknown?

To me, having faith in God or a higher source, being baptised was a way to have peace of mind, that if he did die suddenly, his spirit would be taken care of.

To this day, I would class Victor as having atheist tendencies. He has biblical knowledge, but it is not devout or religious in any way.

If A.I.D.S. comes from denying love, suppressed rage or blocking love, then the affect it has on the spirit is that it can become detached or separate from the mind and body.

This also seems to happen just before people pass away or pass over. Spirit is energy or the essence of the person. It cannot be created or destroyed. In my observations and life experience, having had many relatives pass on and an awareness of past lives, the spirit energy appears to continue on.

I believe that's why Victor appeared to have a rebirth, when he survived his first anaphylactic reaction. He also exhibited babyish gestures immediately after the rebirth like rocking on his back, kicking his legs, cooing and sucking his thumb.

By teaching him to reattach his spirit to his mind and body, he has gained the will to try life again.

I did this by grounding his spirit in his body, through simply enjoying physical activities, hugging and kissing him and connecting with nature. He went to the beach and built sand castles; hiked through forests and climbed mountains; saw the beauty in nature, by experiencing it and watching documentaries.

When he received his long-awaited puppy, he said that it was the happiest day of his life. Every day since is pure joy.

Never underestimate the power of love, joy and contentment a pet can give. Dogs aren't called man's best friend for nothing!

REUNITING DIVINE LOVE AND WILL

'From the beginning we are enlightened energy beings blessed with a sound, basic mind.'

When a person gives up attachment to the separation of the Spirit (Divine Love) and the Soul (Will), they let go of suffering. It is their responsibility to receive God (Golden Original Design) energy and connect the Spirit and Will, by listening and following their own destiny. (Starlight, 2006)

By believing that they can manifest what they will, anything is possible in life, once they put their thought energy to focusing on it. By putting out to the Universe what they want and letting go of the how, when, where and why, manifestation will occur, at some point in time.

It can be anything in the physical, emotional, mental or spiritual realm and sometimes, when they least expect it.

By connecting and balancing the subconscious and conscious mind, it is possible to create, at any given moment.

When enlightenment is grounded in the temple of the body, the soul is healed.

Victor believes he is healed.

I told him that if he believes he is, then he is.

At age thirteen, on his own volition, Victor went to the local Mall after school, without his Epi-Pen. He bought a hazelnut chocolate bar and ate it in its entirety. There was no reaction. . .

THEORIES

'Theories are just someone's notion whether educated or not, until they are proven or disproved.'

At one moment in time, people believed that the Earth was flat. That if someone sailed to the edge of the ocean, their ship would fall off.

There was also a theory, that the Earth was the centre of the Universe. If we gave those early Astronomers modern day tools like a Hubble Telescope and a Space Station, their theories may have been very different.

Over the years, working in the microcosm of schools, I have observed many people, who have various allergies, with varying degrees of reactions.

None of these theories are proven or disproved, as they are governed by personality traits and positions in the family. To date, I am not aware of any studies being done, in this area of psychology.

However, in reading them, they may strike a chord, when observing your own child or yourself, if you are an adult with a nut allergy. If so, this may help you identify triggers to anaphylactic reactions and help you to parent differently, to lessen or eliminate it all together.

I've also observed, that fear of the Epi-Pen Junior/ Epi-Pen injection, often escalates the release of adrenaline and nor-adrenaline from endocrine glands in the body. This appears to slow down the anaphylactic reaction and gives the child the energy to fight being injected.

Even though, it is frustrating for the person trying to perform First Aid, it gives the paramedics a little more time to get there. It is also important to restrain the child if necessary before the auto-injection is given. That way, it won't accidentally misfire or pop out before a full metered dose has been expelled into their body.

That said, I'll be looking at three different reactions to nuts: Airborne; Touch; and Ingestion.

AIRBORNE REACTION TO NUTS

'Ultimate fear is ultimate power when in out of control situations.'

I met a man once named, Oscar. Oscar had a phlegmatic, flamboyant personality. He often over-reacted to situations, no matter how minor. This reaction tended to draw lots of attention, or repelled people with equal intensity.

Oscar lived alone, was a twin and was raised by a dominant, abusive father. His twin was an exceptionally high achiever.

As soon as Oscar entered a room and smelled a whiff of roasted peanuts, he would have an anaphylactic reaction. An Epi-Pen administered pronto, he was transported to hospital by paramedics.

The pay-off was masses amounts of caring attention by hospital staff and everyone with whom he came in contact, the next day at his workplace.

My theory is that when Oscar was a child, his mind found a way to avoid abuse from his father. Perhaps, he was allergic to his father. Perhaps, being the second born twin, he wasn't able to compete with the twin, who coped with the abuse by excelling at everything. Perhaps, he received more attention by having an anaphylactic reaction, or received less physical abuse, because his health was more fragile.

Whatever his initial thought pattern, to cause such an immediate and violent reaction, it gave him ultimate power and control over life and death.

Recently, three ladies were in a room. One lady was eating Peanut Satay. She could hear Oscar's sharp, quick footsteps marching towards us and yelled out an urgent warning to him to stay away.

Distracted, Oscar was talking with another gentleman. He continued to walk into the room, collected some paperwork on the far wall and walked out. No reaction!

I met his eyes, before he exited. There was no fear in them. At that moment, the airborne reaction depended on his thought patterns. Perhaps, the audience wasn't big enough or important enough for him to stage the whole drama or simply, there was no fear in his mind at the time.

Two months on, Oscar is now calm and rational. There has been no more anaphylactic reactions. He has also met a loving partner and doesn't live alone anymore. He loves and nurtures himself, has followed his heart and is happy and content.

TOUCH REACTION TO NUTS

'Strong fear creates a fight or flight reaction when someone is aware of their allergy but has no personal growth or knowledge on how to live their lives happily.'

I met a lady once named Gertrude. Gertrude had a melancholic, nervous personality. She would scream and pull tantrums, if she didn't get her own way. She suffered from stress easily, was very demanding and high-strung.

Gertrude was allergic to almonds. If she found out that she'd touched anything with almonds in it, she would have a meltdown even before it touched her lips. Though she knew that almonds are often used in cakes, pastries, Chinese food and cookies, she would choose to touch them without asking what's in them first. Why? Did she forget? Perhaps, she was suffering from stress and wanted a way out of her situation/ job?

The lady with whom she worked was pregnant. She also wanted to be pregnant, but her stress was preventing it from happening.

Later, a stress burnout enabled her to flee her situation. A sea change and a stint at home enabled her to fall pregnant.

By choosing to have anaphylactic reactions, she could get her own way and time away from her job.

Was her original thought pattern that she didn't want to grow up and take responsibility for her own actions? I wondered.

Nine months later, she is happily staying at home and raising adorable twins. She is calmer and has the time to take better care of herself. Her diet and digestive system has also improved.

INGESTION REACTION TO NUTS

'Mild fear induces a mild reaction when someone doesn't believe or understand their allergy.'

I once met a lady named April. April had a Choleric, cheerful personality. She was enthusiastic, full of energy and multi-talented.

April only had anaphylactic reactions to ingestion of whole walnuts. Ground walnuts in a cake for example didn't create any reaction in her body at all.

April had many hobbies and was very fit. She loved life and nothing really bothered her. April had moved away from her family in Europe where she had previously felt stifled and unable to be whom she was. She also felt the school system there was stifling her children's education.

Now in a country where her own and her children's educational needs were met, she was content and now brims with happiness.

Was the original thought pattern that she didn't want to continue in such a stifling environment? It's a possibility.

EASY FAMILY DINNERS

'In the 60's, dinner was called, 'A square meal '- meat and three types of vegetables.'

During the first year of living with someone in the family with a nut allergy, I made forty-two different meals per week.

It was exhausting thinking up and preparing two separate menus - one for the family and one for Victor.

As I began to work outside the home four days per week, I realised that I had to simplify how I was preparing meals and melding what Victor ate with the rest of the family.

I decided to make toast with butter and Cheesy bite - a spread of Vegemite and cheese for breakfast on week days, have an eat-what-you-like breakfast on Saturday and make pancakes with butter and honey on Sunday.

For school lunches, I would prepare them the night before and both my children would have basically the same thing - Sanitarium Up & Go's; Fruit Juice Poppas; Cheese and Bacon Rolls or Ham sandwiches; Rice Bars; Cheese sticks; Tiny Teddies; Arnott's Crackers; and tubs of fruit or Jelly and Fruit Tubs. All with a bottle of purified water.

For snacks, the boys could go to the pantry or fridge and have whatever they felt like - small tins of spaghetti or baked beans; small packets of chips; biscuits/ cookies; muffins; ice-cream; toast or cereal; yoghurt, fruit, milk and Nesquik or Milo.

For dinner, I would take scoops of whole foods while preparing meals and put them on a plate for Victor. That way, he was basically eating what we were eating and felt part of the family rather than different or special.

There were no extra pots and pans so washing up became easier. Right from the age of two, I taught both my children to do the dishes and they have always taken turns doing them each night. As I was the chief cook, I instilled in my children the importance of giving back or paying it forward.

Both my boys have taken Catering as a subject at High School in Grade 9. Now both cook regularly and I do the washing up.

They have always had paid jobs for pocket money e.g. cleaning the floors, bathtub and vacuuming. The unpaid family jobs were things like alternating washing the dishes; keeping their bedrooms tidy; making their bed once a week after washing the bed linen; putting dirty clothes in the basket provided; and putting rubbish in the bucket in their room; taking out the garbage and putting the bins out for collection once a week.

Victor is one for fairness so he received no special treatment. In fact, often Freddie would pay him to do his jobs!

K.I.S.S. – KEEP IT SIMPLE SUPPERS

'When the family cook also works outside the home, thirty minute meal preparation is greatly appreciated.'

Basically, I worked out a staple weekly menu for suppers which included whole foods that Victor would eat. I would take scoops of each item in the meal when cooked and put it on his plate. Children only have a stomach the size of their fist so they don't need a lot of food to fill them up.

After placing a scoop of rice/ pasta/ bread, steamed or roast vegetables and cooked meat on his plate, I would add the bottled sauces to make tasty meals for the rest of the family.

Victor's favourite and only condiment was tomato sauce/ ketchup. The younger the child is, the more sensitive their taste buds. They often prefer bland food because herbs & spices are too strong for their palate. When they get older, their taste buds are dulled a little. It is then they appreciate and usually ask for tastier food.

Victor ate the same meal at a popular fast food restaurant for four years until he was sick of it. Then, at another popular fast food restaurant, he tried the same meal which was a little spicier. He liked it. This helped especially on travelling holidays when small towns would sometimes have only one type of fast food restaurant.

Back then, fast food restaurants didn't provide allergy information. Due to public demand, this has now changed, so it is easy to find guaranteed nut-free meals that children prefer.

Between the ages of eight and twelve, I followed a regular dinner menu for each week. This kept everyone's taste buds satisfied and provided healthy nutrition especially for working parents and growing children.

DINNER MENU
Sunday - Corned Silverside/ Beef and Roast Vegetables
Monday - Rissoles, Steamed Rice, Carrot and Broccoli
Tuesday - Steamed Rice and Sweet 'n' Sour Chicken with added steamed Carrots and Broccoli
Wednesday - BBQ Chicken, Herb/ Garlic Bread, Frozen Mixed Vegetables (Carrots, Peas & Corn)

Thursday - Rice Pasta and Spaghetti Bolognaise with added steamed Carrots and Broccoli

Friday - Frozen Crumbed Fish and Potato/ Sweet Potato Oven-Baked Fries and Frozen Mixed Vegetables

Saturday – Takeaway/ Takeout

Occasionally, we would have dessert. It would usually consist of ice-cream or yoghurt and/or fruit. I found though, when the children were little, the main meal satisfied them well enough.

Once a week, I would buy a packet of Boysenberry Drumsticks to share with the family. This ice-cream was sprinkled with chocolate instead of nuts. Now, they have Mint and Strawberry which also are nut-free.

DAILY HEALTHY AND BALANCED DIET

A variety of organic, whole foods eaten daily is the ultimate goal for optimum health. With children especially fussy eaters, I began looking at a healthy and balanced diet as being over a week rather than each day.

Sometimes, children aren't hungry. Some like to eat three set meals a day, others like to graze all day. Each child has a unique metabolism. The most important thing is for children to eat when they are hungry and not overeat because they are being forced to finish everything on their plate. More often than not, a child's stomach is only as big as their fist.

When my siblings and I were younger, we were minded for a period of time by our Uncle Jonah when our mother was ill in hospital. Not having any children of his own, every night, he would place big mounds of mashed potato on our plate. Uncle Jonah expected us to eat everything on our plate. After he left the room, when we were full, we would scrape the potato off our plates and out the kitchen window.

After three months, Uncle Jonah found a huge mound of potato in the garden. His temper flared and he left. There was no way we could have eaten that much potato along with the other food on our plates but he wouldn't listen to us.

We were grateful that Uncle Jonah was there during that difficult time because our father always came home from work late. When we were adults, we had the opportunity to thank him for looking after us.

THE IMPORTANT ROLE OF JUNK FOOD

When I grew up, mothers stayed home and saw to taking care of the house and family. They cooked the evening meals and often baked cakes, puddings and biscuits/ cookies. Fathers brought home the bacon and looked after the car, the lawn and the garden.

Nowadays, often both Mum and Dad work outside the home. Other people are paid to do everything from car and house cleaning, to minding the children, to mowing the lawn and tidying the garden.

Fast foods and foods high in sugar, fat and salt, commonly known as Junk Food, are heavily advertised and marketed. They are readily available and children are aware of them from a very young age.

Many birthday parties for young children are held at Fast Food Venues. To totally remove all junk food from your child's diet, especially when they see other children enjoying them at school can create a feeling that they are deprived or missing out. This can subsequently make the child crave them.

I believe it is better to keep a little of the Junk Food in their diet. I found many foods that Victor could have safely and he was satisfied with a treat every now and then.

I found by having takeaway/ takeout once a week, it gave him something to look forward to and me a much needed break from cooking.

As Victor became a teenager and wanted to hang out at the Mall with his friends, food was often consumed in the Food Court, in the Cinema, Bowling Alley or Gaming Arcade. After years of knowing what he could eat safely, the transition to be confident in his teenage independence was simple and easy. To stop him from socialising in this way like most other teenagers was ludicrous. Having an overprotective parent hovering over his shoulder was not an option!

To me, the importance of Victor growing into a confident, independent adult was paramount.

CONCLUSION

'Life is a wondrous journey. The knowledge we gain through our experiences creates the wisdom we pass on to future generations.'

HEAL, HEALING, HEALED

On October 26th, 2012, Victor returned to his original Allergy Specialist at fourteen years of age. He was given a skin prick test.

The Allergy Specialist pronounced that Victor had healed from most of his food and environmental allergies. In seven years, he was now not allergic to hazelnuts or sesame seeds. He had a minimal reaction to peanuts and almonds. The Brazil nut reaction was slightly stronger due to no foods containing this particular nut except packets of the whole nut.

Victor immediately ate chocolate biscuits he'd been dying to taste and Nutella - a chocolate hazelnut spread. The slingshot effect - he said that he wanted to eat the whole world out of Nutella! The pure joy on his face was a sight to behold. It made my heart sing knowing all our hard work had made a difference to the rest of his life.

The Allergy Specialist said that Victor had a good chance of outgrowing all of his allergies by adulthood. Surprisingly, he also didn't charge us for the consultation. He was very pleased to see him and shook his hand. It made me wonder had any of his other patient's returned.

He also informed us that there is a series of injections people with anaphylactic reactions to nuts can have which negates the life-threatening effects of nut allergy. At the writing of this book, it is still in the clinical trial stage.

Determined to be totally cured, Victor returned to the Naturopath a month later for a check-up. Again, the Naturopath put Victor on a course of homeopathic drops to desensitise him from the last of his allergies. When the desensitisation was complete, I waited the required four days before testing him with small amounts of nuts.

On January 2nd, 2013, I wiped a small amount of peanut butter on Victor's lower lip. There was no reaction.

The next morning, I wiped a small amount of Almond, Cashew and Brazil nut Paste on Victor's lower lip. Immediately, he ate some of it. There was a slight reaction - wheezing; the whites of his eyes turned red; and his nose itched. After two minutes, all signs and symptoms disappeared.

Anaphylaxis didn't occur. His immune system had tolerated the nut protein. However, Victor was moody, angry and grumpy, so I gave him some Australian Bush Flower Essence - Abund to clear his negativity.

The next day, Victor expressed his feelings and let me know that his moodiness was due to losing five computer games in a row, not from any fear that I thought may have been attached to his moodiness.

Soon after, Victor returned to the Naturopath who gave him some Spinal Tapping to clear the remaining nut allergies. During the visit, Victor had an epiphany. He fully believed that the treatment had worked.

On January 11th, 2013, the day after Victor's 15th birthday, once again, I wiped a small amount of Almond, Cashew and Brazil Nut Paste on his lower lip.

There was no reaction . . . Victor has now fully healed himself from all his anaphylactic allergies. He is a confident, independent young man who can live the rest of his life well.

When Victor returned to his Doctor, I mentioned that Victor hadn't had an anaphylactic reaction to the nut paste. The Doctor immediately asked for a Blood Test which Victor decided to have. The Blood Tests results showed that the nut protein antibodies were still in his blood stream. The Doctor was surprised and couldn't explain why anaphylaxis hadn't occurred. I believe that the antibodies have been altered enough, so they do not recognise and attack when nut protein enters the body. I believe only further investigation into the microbiological make-up of the antibody's cellular structure will provide the answer. Scientists have discovered that Telomeres which cap individual strands of DNA can shorten and disappear. Telomeres play an important part in cell reproduction and prevent union with other cells if altered. Hence, if the Telomeres have been altered in Victor's antibodies, they may not reproduce or connect with a nut protein when it enters his biological system. At the time of publication, Victor's Doctor wasn't prepared to investigate my theory. But another Scientist or Allergist may want to prove or disprove this theory in the future.

However, Victor is rewarded with good health and is enjoying his life to the full. I feel it is better to heal the whole person, not just the physical aspects, don't you?

APPENDIX

Though home-made or home-cooked food is best for someone with a nut allergy, sometimes, it is not practical or convenient in the modern world for this to occur one hundred percent of the time.

In today's modern world, families come in many configurations. Living conditions are often governed by the culture of the country in which people live and their financial capacity. Many parents and carers are also managing small businesses or working outside the home besides raising a family. Therefore, processed foods have become commonly part of our diets.

Here is a list of Nut-Free Processed Foods that I use. You may find more in the country that you live or know more that you prefer.

LIST OF NUT-FREE PROCESSED FOODS

BREADS & CEREALS

- ✓ White & Wholemeal Bread
- ✓ Pita Bread
- ✓ White & Wholemeal Rolls without sesame seeds on top
- ✓ Cheese & Bacon Rolls
- ✓ Herb & Garlic Bread without sesame seeds on top
- ✓ Raisin Bread
- ✓ Pancakes & Pikelets
- ✓ Crackers & Cheese
- ✓ Cakes & various Biscuits/ Cookies without added nuts
- ✓ Cereals without added nuts, Porridge
- ✓ Rice-based muesli bars
- ✓ Pasta-based easy meals
- ✓

MEATS & MEAT PRODUCTS

- ✓ Sliced ham, pork, chicken
- ✓ Ham & Pineapple/ Hawaiian Pizza
- ✓ Frozen Lasagne, Cannelloni
- ✓ Nachos & Tacos (mince- or Chicken-based)
- ✓ Frozen Crumbed Fish
- ✓ Country-style sausages (check labelling)

- ✓ Cheerios
- ✓ Salmon Dip
- ✓ Meat pies & sausage rolls
- ✓

FRUIT & VEGETABLES

- ✓ Pasties
- ✓ Chinese ready-made sauces
- ✓ Italian ready-made sauces
- ✓ Vegetable Dips
- ✓ Coleslaw
- ✓ Pasta Salad
- ✓ Ready-made mashed potatoes & whole baby potatoes with herbs & butter
- ✓ Frozen Mixed Vegetables
- ✓ Popcorn
- ✓ Tubs of fruit
- ✓ Tubs of fruit & Jelly/ Jello
- ✓ Tubes of fruit
- ✓ Tubes of fruit & yoghurt
- ✓ Frozen berries, fruit yoghurt & sorbets
- ✓ Small fruit juices in sealed containers
- ✓ Dried fruit & fruit cubes
- ✓ Fruit sticks
- ✓ Small boxes of sultanas &/ or sultanas with other fruits
- ✓ Fruit pies & tarts
- ✓ Pavlova
- ✓ Vegetable soups
- ✓

DAIRY PRODUCTS

- ✓ Plain & Fruit Yoghurt without nuts
- ✓ Flavoured milk in sealed containers
- ✓ Milk with added powdered flavourings
- ✓ Yoghurt coated sultanas
- ✓ Frozen yoghurt
- ✓ Ice-cream (without nuts) N.B.* Avoid buying ice-cream from ice-creameries as there may be cross-contamination from multiple utensils being stored in the same water container.
- ✓ Ice-cream cake (Great for birthdays!)

- ✓ Small amounts of cheese in all shapes in sealed packaging
- ✓ Cheese dip & crackers
- ✓ Plain chocolate & chocolate bars without nuts
- ✓

FATS & OILS

- ✓ Potato chips & various savoury snacks (check labelling)
- ✓ Canola oil
- ✓ Sunflower oil
- ✓ Vegetable oil
- ✓ Olive oil with or without garlic
- ✓ Butter
- ✓ Margarine (except nut-based types - check labelling)
- ✓ Check what oil all foods bought outside the home are cooked in. Avoid blended or mixed oils and palm/ coconut oil.
- ✓ Plain & whipped cream
- ✓ Sour light cream
- ✓ Custards & Blanc mange
- ✓ White and Cheese sauce
- ✓ Gravy (check labelling)
- ✓

MISCELLANEOUS

- ✓ Sports drinks with electrolytes
- ✓ Natural fruit lollies
- ✓ Peppermints
- ✓ Chewing or Bubblegum
- ✓ Soft Drinks/ Sodas
- ✓ Bottled water

N.B.* This list is meant as a guide and is in no way exhaustive or specific. It is meant to provide ideas for variety in a healthy diet that is made up of many home-made, wholesome meals. It is also helpful when making up children's lunches or when out and about enjoying life.
ALWAYS CHECK LABELLING FOR PEACE OF MIND AND PLEASE MAKE TIME TO WRITE YOUR OWN LISTS OF FOODS THAT YOUR CHILD LIKES & PREFERS.

LIST OF PROCESSED FOODS THAT MAY CONTAIN TRACES OF NUTS

Many processed foods are made in factories that use equipment that processes tree nuts or products that contain a variety of nuts and sesame seeds. By choosing products that are made in countries that have strict health laws and policies, if the products don't actually contain nuts or sesame seeds in them, they are in general are safe to eat. Equipment is cleaned thoroughly after each type of product is made and airborne traces would be negligible.

The following products are labelled that they may contain traces of nuts by law but may not have any in them or cause a reaction.

They are:
- Muesli Bars
- Breakfast Cereals
- Frozen Savoury Dishes especially Chinese & Indian style
- Frozen Meat Pies & Quiches
- Chocolate Bars
- Biscuits/ Cookies
- Cakes & Slices
- Bread & Bread Rolls
- Sausage meats
- Sauces & Gravies

N.B.* It is your choice whether to give bits of these foods.

REFERENCES AND RESOURCES

BOOKS

PERFECT HEALTH - Deepak Chopra MD - Bantam Books, 1990

THE SEVEN SPIRITUAL LAWS OF SUCCESS FOR PARENTS - Guiding Your Children To Success and Fulfilment - Deepak Chopra - Rider, Ebury Press, Random House, 1997

AGELESS BODY TIMELESS MIND - Deepak Chopra MD - Crown Publications, 1998

HOW TO KNOW GOD - Deepak Chopra - Rider, Ebury Press, Random House, 2000

GROW YOUNGER LIVE LONGER - Deepak Chopra MD with David Simon MD - Rider, Ebury Press, Random House, 2001

QUANTUM HEALING - Deepak Chopra MD - Conari Press U.S., 2011

YOU CAN HEAL YOUR LIFE - Louise L. Hay - Specialist Publications, 1984

THE BODY IS THE BAROMETER OF THE SOUL SO BE YOUR OWN DOCTOR 2 - Annette Noontil - Brumby Books, 1994

YOUR CHILD'S DEVELOPMENT FROM BIRTH TO ADOLESCENCE - Richard Lansdown & Marjorie Walker - Angus & Robertson, Harper Collins Publishers, 1992

GREEN BABIES - Dr Penney Stanway - Random Century Group, 1990

RAISING A SON, PARENTS AND THE MAKING OF A HEALTHY MAN - Don Elium & Jeanne Elium - Beyond Words Publishing, 1992

RAISING A DAUGHTER, PARENTS AND THE MAKING OF A HEALTHY DAUGHTER - Don Elium & Jeanne Elium - Beyond Words Publishing, 1992

BABIES - Dr Christopher Green & Dr Hilary Green - Simon & Schuster, 1988

TODDLER TAMING - Dr Christopher Green - Doubleday, 1990

BEYOND TODDLERDOM - Dr Christopher Green - Doubleday Book, Transworld Publishers, Random House, 2000

TOXIC PARENTS - Dr Susan Forward - Bantam Books, 1989

EVERYWOMAN - Derek Llewellyn-Jones - Faber and Faber Limited, 1971

EVERYMAN - Derek Llewellyn-Jones - Oxford University Press, 1981

THE INNER MAN - Peter O'Connor - Pan Macmillan Publishers, 1993

THE WOMAN'S GUIDE TO HOMEOPATHY - Dr Andrew Lockie & Dr Nicola Geddes - BCA, 1992
HIDDEN DANGERS - Lillian Reekie - Health & Wealth Solutions, 2003
AUSTRALIAN WELLBEING SURVIVAL LOW-COST, LOW-ALLERGY COOKBOOK - Sally Hammond & Karin Cutter - The Wellspring Publishers Pty Ltd, 1991
THE COMPLETE NATURAL HEALTH CONSULTANT - Michael van Straten - Angus & Robertson Publishers, 1987
JOY - Jennifer Starlight - Joshua Books, 2006
THE HEART OF LOVE - Dr John F. Demartini - Hay House Inc., 2007
BABY SIGNS - Debbie Frank - Vermillion Arrow, Ebury Press, Random House, 1995
CHILD SIGNS - Dodie & Allan Edmands - Hutchinson Group (Aust.) Pty Ltd, 1979
STAR SIGNS - Linda Goodman - Macmillan, Pan Books, 1987
THE NEW ASTROLOGY - Suzanne White - Macmillan, Pan Books, 1986
THE 7 HABITS OF HIGHLY EFFECTIVE TEENS - Sean Covey - Fireside, Simon & Schuster, 1998
THE 6 MOST IMPORTANT DECISIONS YOU'LL EVER MAKE, A GUIDE FOR TEENS - Sean Covey - Fireside, Simon & Schuster, 2006
PEACEFUL WARRIOR - Dan Millman - H J Kramer New World Library, 2010
INSPIRATION: YOUR ULTIMATE CALLING – Dr Wayne W. Dyer - Hay House, 2006
BECOMING ENLIGHTENED - His Holiness the Dalai Lama - Rider, Ebury Press Publishing, 2009

FILMS
THE DEEP END OF THE OCEAN - 1999 Sony Pictures Entertainment
THE SECRET - 2006 Prime Time Productions
WHAT THE BLEEP DO WE KNOW? - 2004 Hopscotch Entertainment
YOU CAN HEAL YOUR LIFE THE MOVIE - 2007 Hay House Inc.

WEBSITES

www.allergy.org.au
www.parenthood.com
www.epiclub.com.au
www.epiclub.co.nz

N.B. **A vast array of Classical Music in F Sharp can be easily accessed on *Youtube*. Playing this classical piano music to babies and toddlers whilst awake or asleep would be most beneficial as the language part in the brain is developing.

ABOUT THE AUTHOR

Natalia Elder is a caring and compassionate woman. First and foremost, she provides a loving, nurturing home for her husband, two children and pets. She enjoys yoga and meditation, live theatre, going to the cinema, walking the dog, connecting with Mother Earth, reading, writing romance novels and Hollywood screenplays, and making the occasional short film.

She is qualified in many aspects of life including: School Dental Therapy; Dental Assisting; Education Support; First Aid; and is a Psychic Counsellor, Reiki Master and Diamond Light Practitioner.

Having studied a vast array of psychology, astrology, philosophies, religions, creative writing & Natural Therapies in her own time, she has a balanced and positive look on life. 'Anything is possible for the good of all' is her mantra.

Her purpose in life is to help all living things on the planet.

Follow Victor's continuing life journey on Facebook Page: Facebook.com/my child is not a nut allergy. His Nan shares wholesome, nut-free recipes especially for children with a secret ingredient. Please feel free to like the Victor's Facebook Page to receive notification when a new post appears.

Natalia would love to hear your stories of your children healing themselves from anaphylaxis, or if you require assistance with Astrological Birth Charts, Reiki and/or Diamond Light Healing on all levels – physical, emotional, mental and spiritual – consultations are available.

Initial contact can be made via email: nataliaelder@outlook.com.

Skype calls will be arranged for those people living in other global locations.

FINAL WORDS OF LOVE

Believe and love yourself. Teach kindness, respect and compassion for all peoples, animals and Mother Nature. Find the love and beauty in all conscious beings. Find the love in your heart and enjoy living in it. Making passionate decisions with your heart are your true pathways. Thought patterns of the mind often get in the way and will tell you all things right and wrong with your heart choices. Within your heart resides your soul and it's the soul's journey which is most important to you in this lifetime. Use integrity as your guide to what's right and wrong for you. It will keep you on track to reach your heart's desires and goals, especially when your desire is to heal yourself or your child from anaphylactic nut allergy.

INDEX

NOTES

Printed in Great Britain
by Amazon

38195483R00067